Courageous in Chaos: How to Find Calm in Turbulent Times

Benjamin Drath

Published by Benjamin Drath, 2024.

COURAGEOUS IN CHAOS: HOW TO FIND CALM IN TURBULENT TIMES

First edition. March 29, 2024.

ISBN: 979-8224474417

Written by Benjamin Drath.

Table of Contents

Opening:

In the tempest of life, where chaos reigns and uncertainty lurks around every corner, it is easy to feel overwhelmed, lost in the tumultuous currents that threaten to pull us under. Turbulent times test our resolve, challenging our inner strength and resilience. Yet, within the storm, there exists a sanctuary of peace, a bastion of courage where the brave find solace amidst the chaos.

Welcome to "Courageous in Chaos: How to Find Calm in Turbulent Times". In these pages, we embark on a journey of self-discovery and empowerment, where we navigate the choppy waters of adversity with courage and grace. Drawing upon ancient wisdom and modern insights, this book serves as a guiding light, illuminating the path towards inner tranquility and steadfastness.

As the world spins ever faster, and the tempests of life grow fiercer, it becomes imperative to cultivate the courage to stand tall in the face of adversity, to embrace the chaos with an unwavering spirit. Through the stories of those who have weathered the storms and emerged stronger, and through the timeless teachings of resilience and fortitude, we learn that true calm is not found in the absence of chaos, but rather in the courage to confront it head-on.

So, let us embark on this journey together, dear reader, as we discover the power of bravery in the midst of chaos, and learn to find peace in the most turbulent of times. For within each of us lies the strength to weather any storm, and the wisdom to find calm amidst the chaos.

Chapter 1: Introduction.

———

I n the tumultuous journey of life, navigating through the unpredictable storms and turbulent seas is an inevitable reality. Yet, amidst the chaos, there exists a profound imperative – the quest to find calm in the midst of the tempest. This introductory chapter serves as a beacon of light, guiding us towards understanding the significance of tranquility in chaos and the transformative power of courage in turbulent times.

Why is it important to find calm in chaos?

Chaos is an ever-present force in our lives, manifesting in various forms such as uncertainty, adversity, and upheaval. It disrupts our equilibrium, triggers stress, and threatens to overwhelm us. In the face of chaos, finding calm is not merely a luxury but a necessity for our well-being and resilience.

Firstly, calmness acts as a shield against the ravages of stress. When we remain composed amidst chaos, we are better equipped to handle challenges with clarity and focus. Rather than succumbing to panic or anxiety, we can approach problems with a sense of serenity, enabling us to make rational decisions and navigate through obstacles more effectively.

Moreover, finding calm in chaos fosters emotional stability and mental resilience. It provides a sanctuary of peace amidst the storm, allowing us to process our emotions with equanimity and maintain our psychological balance. Instead of being swept away by the turbulent currents of despair or frustration, we can anchor ourselves in a state of inner tranquility, emerging from adversity stronger and more resilient than before.

Furthermore, calmness is conducive to creativity and innovation. In moments of stillness, our minds are free to wander, explore new possibilities, and generate innovative solutions to complex problems. By cultivating a calm demeanor amidst chaos, we unlock the creative potential within us, transcending the limitations imposed by external turmoil.

Ultimately, finding calm in chaos is essential for fostering a sense of inner peace and well-being. It allows us to cultivate a deeper connection with ourselves, transcend the external distractions and turmoil, and tap into the inherent serenity that resides within us. In the words of Ralph Waldo Emerson, "Nothing can bring you peace but yourself."

How can courage help us in turbulent times?

Courage is the indomitable spirit that enables us to confront adversity with resilience, to face uncertainty with conviction, and to embrace change with steadfastness. In turbulent times, courage is not merely a virtue but a lifeline that sustains us amidst the raging storms of life.

First and foremost, courage empowers us to confront our fears and uncertainties head-on. Rather than succumbing to the paralyzing grip of fear, courageous individuals stand tall in the face of adversity, refusing to be intimidated by the challenges that confront them. They draw strength from within, harnessing their inner fortitude to confront obstacles with unwavering determination.

Moreover, courage instills a sense of resilience and perseverance in the face of setbacks. It enables us to bounce back from failure, to learn from our mistakes, and to press forward with renewed determination. Instead of being deterred by obstacles, courageous individuals view them as opportunities for growth and self-improvement, channeling their setbacks into stepping stones towards success.

Furthermore, courage inspires others to follow suit, creating a ripple effect of positive change and transformation. When we witness acts of courage in others, we are inspired to emulate their example, to overcome our own fears and limitations, and to embrace the challenges that lie ahead. In this way, courage becomes a catalyst for collective empowerment and societal progress.

Ultimately, courage is the cornerstone of resilience, the bedrock upon which our inner strength and fortitude are built. It is the unwavering belief in our ability to overcome adversity, the refusal to be defined by our circumstances, and the determination to forge our own path amidst the turbulence of life.

In conclusion, finding calm in chaos and cultivating courage in turbulent times are not mere abstract ideals but essential pillars of personal growth and resilience. As we embark on this journey of self-discovery and empowerment, let us embrace the transformative power of calmness and courage, and emerge from the storms of life stronger, wiser, and more resilient than ever before.

Chapter 2: Understanding the nature of chaos.

―――

In the vast tapestry of existence, chaos is an intrinsic and omnipresent force that shapes the very fabric of our reality. It is a phenomenon characterized by disorder, unpredictability, and complexity, defying our attempts to impose order and control. To truly comprehend the nature of chaos is to embark on a journey of introspection and exploration, delving into the depths of the unknown and unraveling the mysteries of existence.

What is chaos?

At its core, chaos is a state of disorder and randomness, devoid of any discernible pattern or structure. It is the antithesis of order, challenging our fundamental assumptions about the predictability and stability of the universe. From the chaotic swirl of subatomic particles to the turbulent currents of the cosmos, chaos permeates every level of existence, shaping the evolution of galaxies, stars, and planets.

However, chaos is not merely a destructive force but also a creative one, giving rise to the infinite diversity and complexity of the cosmos. In the chaotic interplay of natural processes, new forms emerge, old structures crumble, and novel patterns emerge from the primordial chaos. It is this dynamic interplay of order and chaos that drives the process of evolution, shaping the destiny of life itself.

Moreover, chaos is inherently nonlinear and sensitive to initial conditions, exhibiting a phenomenon known as "sensitivity to initial conditions." This means that even small changes in the starting conditions of a chaotic system can lead to drastically different outcomes, amplifying the unpredictability and complexity of chaotic phenomena. This sensitivity to initial conditions is exemplified by the famous "butterfly effect," where the flapping of a butterfly's wings in one part of the world can potentially trigger a chain reaction of events leading to a tornado in another part of the world.

Why do we experience turbulent times?

Turbulent times are the manifestation of chaos in human affairs, characterized by upheaval, uncertainty, and instability. They arise from a myriad of interconnected factors, including social, economic, political, and environmental forces, which conspire to create a perfect storm of chaos and disruption.

One of the primary causes of turbulent times is the inherent complexity and interconnectedness of modern society. In an increasingly globalized world, the ripple effects of economic crises, political upheavals, and environmental disasters can spread rapidly across borders, creating a domino effect of instability and uncertainty. Moreover, rapid technological advancements and social changes further exacerbate the complexity of the modern world, introducing new challenges and uncertainties into our lives.

Furthermore, turbulent times often arise from the clash of competing interests and ideologies, as different groups and individuals vie for power, resources, and influence. These conflicts can escalate into full-blown crises, destabilizing entire societies and plunging them into chaos and turmoil.

Additionally, turbulent times may also be fueled by natural disasters, such as earthquakes, hurricanes, and pandemics, which disrupt the normal functioning of society and pose existential threats to human civilization. These catastrophic events not only cause immediate suffering and devastation but also have long-term repercussions that reverberate throughout the fabric of society.

Ultimately, turbulent times are a natural consequence of living in a chaotic and ever-changing world. While they may bring hardship and adversity, they also present opportunities for growth, transformation, and renewal. By understanding the nature of chaos and its impact on our lives, we can learn to navigate through turbulent times with resilience, adaptability, and courage, emerging stronger and more resilient than before.

Chapter 3: The significance of courage.

———

In the labyrinth of life's trials and tribulations, courage stands as a beacon of hope, guiding us through the darkest of times and empowering us to overcome our fears. It is a virtue revered by poets, philosophers, and warriors alike, embodying the indomitable spirit of resilience and determination. In this chapter, we delve into the profound significance of courage, exploring its essence, its manifestations, and its transformative power in helping us find calm amidst the storms of life.

What is courage?

Courage is a multifaceted virtue that transcends mere bravery or fearlessness. It is the inner strength that enables us to confront our deepest fears and insecurities, to persevere in the face of adversity, and to stand firm in our convictions even when the odds are stacked against us. At its core, courage is not the absence of fear but rather the willingness to act in spite of fear, to defy the whispers of doubt and uncertainty and forge ahead with unwavering resolve.

Courage manifests itself in myriad forms, from the quiet courage of everyday heroes who perform acts of kindness and compassion in the face of adversity, to the bold courage of trailblazers who challenge the status quo and pave the way for change. It is the courage of a parent standing up for their child, the courage of a soldier facing the horrors of war, and the courage of an artist baring their soul to the world through their art.

Moreover, courage is not a fixed trait but rather a muscle that can be strengthened and cultivated through practice and perseverance. It requires courage to step outside of our comfort zones, to embrace vulnerability, and to take risks in pursuit of our dreams and aspirations. By facing our fears head-on and pushing past our self-imposed limitations, we unlock the boundless potential within us and emerge stronger, wiser, and more resilient than before.

How can courage help us find calm?

Courage serves as a powerful antidote to fear, offering us the strength and resilience to confront the chaos and uncertainty of life with grace and composure. In times of turmoil and upheaval, it is courage that anchors us amidst the storm, enabling us to find calm in the midst of chaos.

First and foremost, courage empowers us to confront our fears and insecurities head-on, rather than allowing them to dictate our actions and decisions. When we summon the courage to face our fears with conviction and determination, we diminish their power over us and reclaim control over our lives. Instead of being paralyzed by fear, we are emboldened to take decisive action and move forward with confidence and purpose.

Moreover, courage enables us to embrace vulnerability and authenticity, fostering deeper connections with ourselves and others. When we have the courage to be true to ourselves, to express our thoughts and feelings openly and honestly, we cultivate a sense of inner peace and authenticity that transcends the chaos and turmoil of external circumstances. In this state of vulnerability, we find strength, resilience, and a profound sense of calm that emanates from within.

Furthermore, courage fosters a sense of perspective and resilience that enables us to weather the storms of life with grace and equanimity. Instead of being consumed by fear and anxiety, we are able to maintain a sense of calm and clarity, even in the face of adversity. By cultivating a courageous mindset grounded in resilience and determination, we are better equipped to navigate through turbulent times with grace, poise, and resilience.

In conclusion, courage is not merely a virtue but a transformative force that empowers us to find calm amidst the chaos of life. By summoning the courage to confront our fears, embrace vulnerability, and cultivate resilience, we unlock the inner strength and fortitude needed to navigate through life's storms with grace and composure. In the words of Nelson Mandela, "Courage is not the absence of fear, but the triumph over it."

Chapter 4: Self-reflection.

———

In the midst of life's tumultuous storms, amidst the chaos and uncertainty that surrounds us, there exists a sanctuary of stillness and clarity – the realm of self-reflection. In this chapter, we explore the profound importance of self-reflection in turbulent times, and how it serves as a powerful tool for finding calm amidst the tempests of life.

The importance of self-reflection in turbulent times

Turbulent times often leave us feeling overwhelmed and disoriented, buffeted by the winds of change and uncertainty. In the midst of chaos, it is all too easy to lose sight of ourselves, to become disconnected from our innermost thoughts, feelings, and aspirations. Yet, it is precisely in these moments of upheaval that self-reflection becomes indispensable, offering us a lifeline of clarity and perspective amidst the storm.

Self-reflection is the process of turning inward, of delving deep into the recesses of our minds and souls to explore our thoughts, emotions, and beliefs. It is a journey of self-discovery and introspection, where we confront our fears, insecurities, and doubts with courage and compassion. By shining a light into the darkest corners of our being, we gain insight into ourselves, uncovering hidden truths and untapped potentials that lie dormant within us.

Moreover, self-reflection is a powerful tool for personal growth and development, enabling us to learn from our experiences and mistakes, and to chart a course towards a more fulfilling and authentic life. In times of turbulence, self-reflection serves as a compass, guiding us through the labyrinth of uncertainty and change, and helping us navigate towards a brighter and more hopeful future.

Furthermore, self-reflection fosters resilience and emotional well-being, providing us with a sense of inner peace and stability amidst the chaos and turmoil of external circumstances. By cultivating a practice of self-reflection, we learn to cultivate a sense of inner calm and serenity that transcends the chaos and uncertainty of the outside world.

How can we find calm through self-reflection?

Finding calm through self-reflection is a deeply personal and introspective process, unique to each individual. Yet, there are several key principles and practices that can help us harness the power of self-reflection to cultivate a sense of inner peace and tranquility amidst turbulent times.

Firstly, carving out dedicated time and space for self-reflection is essential. In the hustle and bustle of daily life, it can be all too easy to neglect our inner selves, to prioritize external distractions and obligations over our own well-being. Yet, it is precisely during times of chaos and upheaval that we need self-reflection the most. By setting aside regular periods of quiet contemplation, whether through meditation, journaling, or simply sitting in silence, we create a sacred space for self-discovery and introspection.

Moreover, approaching self-reflection with an open and curious mindset is crucial. Rather than seeking to escape from or suppress our thoughts and emotions, we must embrace them with compassion and acceptance. By observing our thoughts and feelings with non-judgmental awareness, we create the conditions for healing and transformation to occur.

Furthermore, practicing gratitude and mindfulness can deepen our self-reflection practice, helping us cultivate a sense of inner peace and contentment amidst the chaos and uncertainty of external circumstances. By focusing on the present moment and acknowledging the blessings and beauty that surround us, we shift our perspective from fear and scarcity to abundance and gratitude.

In conclusion, self-reflection is a potent tool for finding calm amidst the storms of life. By turning inward, exploring our innermost thoughts and feelings with courage and compassion, we gain insight into ourselves, uncover hidden truths, and cultivate a sense of inner peace and tranquility that transcends the chaos and uncertainty of external circumstances. As we navigate through turbulent times, let us remember the transformative power of self-reflection, and embrace it as a guiding light on our journey towards inner healing and wholeness.

Chapter 5: Acceptance and letting go.

———

In the intricate dance of life, there comes a time when we must confront the immutable truth of impermanence – the inevitability of change, loss, and transformation. In this chapter, we delve into the profound significance of acceptance and letting go, exploring why they are essential virtues in navigating the complexities of existence and how they can lead us to find peace amidst the turbulent currents of life.

Why is acceptance important?

Acceptance is the art of embracing reality as it is, without resistance or judgment. It is the willingness to acknowledge and come to terms with the imperfections and uncertainties of life, recognizing that the only constant in life is change. While acceptance may seem passive or resigned, it is, in fact, a deeply empowering act that frees us from the shackles of attachment and suffering.

Firstly, acceptance enables us to find peace amidst the chaos and uncertainty of life. When we resist reality or cling to unrealistic expectations, we set ourselves up for disappointment and frustration. However, when we accept things as they are, we release ourselves from the burden of unmet expectations and open ourselves to the possibility of finding contentment and fulfillment in the present moment.

Moreover, acceptance fosters resilience and emotional well-being. By acknowledging and accepting our own limitations and vulnerabilities, we cultivate a sense of self-compassion and inner strength that enables us to weather the storms of life with grace and equanimity. Instead of being consumed by regret or resentment, we learn to accept the past as it is and focus on creating a brighter future.

Furthermore, acceptance is the gateway to transformation and growth. When we accept reality as it is, we create the space for change and evolution to occur.

Instead of clinging to outdated beliefs or habits, we embrace the opportunity for self-discovery and self-improvement, paving the way for personal and spiritual growth.

How can we learn to let go?

Letting go is the art of releasing attachments and surrendering to the flow of life. It is the process of relinquishing control and allowing things to unfold naturally, without interference or resistance. While letting go may seem daunting or uncomfortable, it is a necessary step on the path to inner peace and liberation.

One of the key principles of letting go is cultivating mindfulness and present-moment awareness. By grounding ourselves in the here and now, we become more attuned to the ever-changing nature of reality and less attached to past regrets or future anxieties. Through practices such as meditation, yoga, or simply being fully present in our daily activities, we learn to let go of the past and future and embrace the richness of the present moment.

Moreover, letting go requires cultivating trust and faith in the inherent wisdom of life. Instead of trying to control or manipulate outcomes, we learn to surrender to the natural flow of life and trust that everything is unfolding exactly as it should. By relinquishing the need to constantly struggle and strive, we find peace and contentment in simply being.

Furthermore, letting go is about releasing attachments and expectations. Whether it's letting go of material possessions, relationships, or limiting beliefs, the act of releasing attachments frees us from the burden of clinging and opens us to the possibility of new beginnings. By detaching ourselves from outcomes and allowing things to unfold organically, we create space for miracles to occur.

In conclusion, acceptance and letting go are essential practices for finding peace and fulfillment in the midst of life's challenges. By accepting reality as it is and learning to let go of attachments and expectations, we free ourselves from the shackles of suffering and open ourselves to the infinite possibilities of life. As we embark on this journey of self-discovery and liberation, may we embrace the transformative power of acceptance and letting go, and find peace amidst the ever-changing currents of existence.

Chapter 6: Cultivating serenity.

———

In the chaotic symphony of life, serenity stands as a rare and precious jewel – a state of inner peace and tranquility that transcends the turmoil and tribulations of the external world. In this chapter, we explore the art of cultivating serenity, delving into the profound significance of this virtue in difficult situations and offering practical exercises to help us nurture a sense of calm amidst the storm.

The art of serenity in difficult situations.

Serenity is not merely the absence of chaos or adversity but rather the ability to remain calm and centered amidst the storms of life. It is a state of inner peace and tranquility that arises from a deep sense of acceptance, surrender, and trust in the inherent wisdom of life. While serenity may seem elusive in the face of difficulty and turmoil, it is, in fact, a potent antidote to the suffering and stress that often accompany challenging situations.

One of the key principles of cultivating serenity is learning to let go of resistance and surrender to the flow of life. Instead of fighting against the currents of change or struggling to control outcomes, we learn to embrace the ebb and flow of existence with grace and equanimity. By relinquishing the need to constantly resist or manipulate reality, we create the space for serenity to emerge naturally.

Moreover, cultivating serenity requires cultivating mindfulness and present-moment awareness. By grounding ourselves in the here and now, we become more attuned to the richness and beauty of the present moment and less consumed by worries or regrets about the past or future. Through practices such as meditation, deep breathing, or simply paying attention to our senses, we cultivate a sense of inner peace and stillness that transcends the chaos and turmoil of external circumstances.

Furthermore, cultivating serenity involves cultivating self-compassion and self-care. In times of difficulty and stress, it is all too easy to neglect our own well-being and prioritize the needs of others. Yet, self-care is not selfish but rather essential for maintaining our physical, emotional, and spiritual health. By prioritizing activities that nourish and replenish us, such as exercise, hobbies, or spending time in nature, we cultivate a sense of inner peace and well-being that radiates outwards to others.

Practical exercises to cultivate serenity.

Mindful breathing: Take a few moments each day to practice mindful breathing, focusing your attention on the sensation of your breath as it enters and leaves your body. Notice the rise and fall of your chest, the rhythm of your breath, and the sensation of air filling your lungs. With each inhale, imagine breathing in calmness and serenity, and with each exhale, imagine releasing tension and stress.

Gratitude journaling: Set aside a few minutes each day to write down three things you are grateful for. They can be big or small, simple or profound – the key is to focus on the blessings and abundance in your life rather than dwelling on what is lacking. By cultivating an attitude of gratitude, you shift your focus from negativity to positivity and create space for serenity to flourish.

Nature immersion: Spend time in nature regularly, whether it's going for a walk in the park, hiking in the mountains, or simply sitting in your backyard. Notice the beauty and tranquility of the natural world around you – the rustling of leaves, the chirping of birds, the gentle sway of trees in the breeze. Allow yourself to be fully present in the moment, immersing yourself in the serenity of nature and allowing it to nourish your soul.

Loving-kindness meditation: Practice loving-kindness meditation to cultivate compassion and goodwill towards yourself and others. Begin by directing loving-kindness towards yourself, repeating phrases such as "May I be happy, may I be healthy, may I be safe, may I be at peace." Then, extend these wishes outward to loved ones, acquaintances, and even those you may have difficulty with. By cultivating feelings of love and compassion, you create a sense of interconnectedness and harmony that fosters serenity.

In conclusion, cultivating serenity is a journey of self-discovery and inner transformation that requires patience, practice, and perseverance. By embracing the art of serenity in difficult situations and committing to practical exercises that nourish our mind, body, and spirit, we can cultivate a deep sense of inner peace and tranquility that sustains us amidst the storms of life. As we embark on this journey, may we remember that true serenity lies not in the absence of difficulty but in our ability to remain calm and centered amidst the chaos and turmoil of existence.

Chapter 7: The power of patience.

———

I n the fast-paced and frenetic world we live in, patience stands as a beacon of strength and resilience – a virtue that enables us to weather the storms of life with grace and equanimity. In this chapter, we explore the profound significance of patience as a virtue and its transformative power in navigating turbulent times. We'll delve into why patience is considered a virtue and offer practical insights on how we can cultivate patience amidst life's uncertainties.

Why is patience a virtue?

Patience is often heralded as a virtue because of its ability to foster inner peace, resilience, and emotional well-being. At its core, patience is the ability to endure hardships and delays with calmness and fortitude, without succumbing to frustration or impatience. It is a virtue that enables us to maintain perspective, stay grounded in the present moment, and respond to challenges with clarity and grace.

Firstly, patience is essential for maintaining healthy relationships and fostering harmony in our interactions with others. In a world where instant gratification is often prized above all else, patience allows us to communicate more effectively, listen attentively, and resolve conflicts with empathy and understanding. By practicing patience, we cultivate deeper connections with others and build stronger, more meaningful relationships.

Moreover, patience is essential for achieving long-term goals and aspirations. In a society that values speed and efficiency, it's easy to become discouraged when progress is slow or setbacks occur. However, patience enables us to stay focused on our objectives, persevere through adversity, and trust in the process of growth and transformation. By cultivating patience, we develop resilience and determination that propels us towards success, despite the obstacles we may encounter along the way.

Furthermore, patience is a key ingredient for cultivating inner peace and emotional well-being. In a world filled with stress and uncertainty, patience allows us to respond to challenges with equanimity, rather than reacting impulsively out of fear or frustration. By cultivating patience, we develop a sense of inner calm and tranquility that enables us to navigate life's ups and downs with grace and resilience.

How can we cultivate patience in turbulent times?

Cultivating patience in turbulent times requires practice, perseverance, and a willingness to embrace discomfort and uncertainty. Here are some practical insights on how we can cultivate patience amidst life's uncertainties:

Practice mindfulness: Mindfulness is the practice of being fully present in the moment, without judgment or attachment. By cultivating mindfulness through practices such as meditation, deep breathing, or mindful walking, we develop greater awareness of our thoughts, emotions, and reactions. This awareness enables us to respond to challenges with patience and equanimity, rather than reacting impulsively out of habit or conditioning.

Cultivate compassion: Compassion is the ability to empathize with the suffering of others and respond with kindness and understanding. By cultivating compassion towards ourselves and others, we develop greater patience and tolerance for the imperfections and shortcomings of ourselves and those around us. This compassionate attitude fosters deeper connections with others and promotes harmony in our relationships.

Set realistic expectations: In a world that often demands instant results and gratification, it's important to set realistic expectations for ourselves and others. By acknowledging that growth and progress take time and effort, we can cultivate patience and perseverance in our pursuit of goals and aspirations. Instead of becoming discouraged by setbacks or delays, we can view them as opportunities for learning and growth.

Practice gratitude: Gratitude is the practice of acknowledging and appreciating the blessings and abundance in our lives, even amidst challenges and difficulties. By cultivating gratitude through practices such as keeping a gratitude journal or expressing appreciation to others, we develop a more positive outlook on life and cultivate patience and resilience in the face of adversity.

In conclusion, patience is a virtue that empowers us to navigate life's uncertainties with grace, resilience, and equanimity. By cultivating patience through mindfulness, compassion, realistic expectations, and gratitude, we develop greater resilience and emotional well-being that enables us to thrive amidst the turbulence of life. As we embrace the power of patience, may we cultivate a deeper sense of inner peace and tranquility that sustains us on our journey towards fulfillment and happiness.

Chapter 8: Emotional intelligence.

———

In the labyrinth of life, where chaos reigns and uncertainty lurks around every corner, emotional intelligence emerges as a guiding light – a beacon of clarity and understanding amidst the turbulence of our emotions. In this chapter, we explore the profound role of emotional intelligence in navigating chaos and offer practical insights on how we can strengthen these essential skills to thrive amidst life's uncertainties.

The role of emotional intelligence in navigating chaos.

Emotional intelligence, often referred to as EQ, is the ability to recognize, understand, and manage our own emotions, as well as the emotions of others. It encompasses a wide range of skills, including self-awareness, self-regulation, empathy, and social skills, all of which are essential for navigating the complexities of human relationships and the challenges of life.

In the face of chaos and uncertainty, emotional intelligence becomes an indispensable tool for maintaining composure, making informed decisions, and fostering resilience. Here are some ways in which emotional intelligence plays a crucial role in navigating chaos:

Self-awareness: Self-awareness is the foundation of emotional intelligence, enabling us to recognize and understand our own emotions, thoughts, and behaviors. In times of chaos, self-awareness allows us to remain grounded amidst the storm, helping us to identify and acknowledge our feelings without becoming overwhelmed by them. By cultivating self-awareness, we gain insight into our triggers and patterns of behavior, empowering us to respond to challenges with clarity and intention.

Self-regulation: Self-regulation is the ability to manage and control our emotions, impulses, and reactions, even in the face of adversity. In chaotic situations, self-regulation enables us to maintain composure and poise, rather than reacting impulsively out of fear or anger. By practicing techniques such as deep breathing, mindfulness, and positive self-talk, we can cultivate greater emotional resilience and self-control, allowing us to navigate through turbulent times with grace and equanimity.

Empathy: Empathy is the ability to understand and share the feelings of others, to see the world through their eyes and connect with them on a deeper level. In chaotic situations, empathy enables us to foster compassion and understanding towards others, even amidst conflict or disagreement. By practicing active listening, perspective-taking, and non-judgmental communication, we can cultivate empathy and build stronger, more meaningful relationships with others.

Social skills: Social skills are the ability to effectively navigate social situations, build rapport with others, and communicate assertively and diplomatically. In times of chaos, social skills enable us to collaborate effectively with others, to resolve conflicts and negotiate solutions, and to build consensus amidst diversity of opinions. By practicing effective communication, conflict resolution, and teamwork, we can leverage our social skills to navigate through turbulent times with grace and resilience.

How can we strengthen our emotional intelligence?

Strengthening our emotional intelligence is a lifelong journey that requires self-awareness, practice, and commitment. Here are some practical insights on how we can cultivate and strengthen our emotional intelligence:

Practice mindfulness: Mindfulness is a powerful tool for cultivating self-awareness and self-regulation, enabling us to observe our thoughts, emotions, and reactions without judgment or attachment. By practicing mindfulness meditation, deep breathing, or other mindfulness techniques, we can develop greater awareness of our inner world and cultivate emotional resilience.

Reflect on your emotions: Take time each day to reflect on your emotions, identifying the triggers and patterns of behavior that influence your thoughts and actions. Journaling can be a helpful tool for exploring your feelings and gaining insight into your emotional landscape. By cultivating a habit of self-reflection, you can deepen your understanding of yourself and strengthen your emotional intelligence.

Cultivate empathy: Cultivate empathy towards yourself and others by practicing active listening, perspective-taking, and compassion. Take time to truly listen to others, seeking to understand their perspective and validate their feelings. Practice putting yourself in their shoes, imagining how they might be feeling and what they might need from you. By cultivating empathy, you can build stronger, more meaningful relationships and enhance your emotional intelligence.

Seek feedback: Seek feedback from others about your emotional intelligence, asking for honest and constructive input about your strengths and areas for growth. Pay attention to how others perceive your communication style, interpersonal skills, and ability to manage emotions. Use this feedback as an opportunity for self-improvement, reflecting on ways you can enhance your emotional intelligence in your interactions with others.

Practice emotional regulation: Practice techniques for managing and regulating your emotions, such as deep breathing, progressive muscle relaxation, and positive self-talk. When faced with challenging situations, take a moment to pause and breathe deeply, allowing yourself to center and ground before responding. Practice reframing negative thoughts and beliefs into more positive and empowering ones, fostering a sense of inner calm and resilience.

In conclusion, emotional intelligence is a vital skill set for navigating chaos and uncertainty, enabling us to maintain composure, foster resilience, and build stronger, more meaningful relationships. By cultivating self-awareness, self-regulation, empathy, and social skills, we can strengthen our emotional intelligence and thrive amidst life's uncertainties. As we embark on this journey of self-discovery and growth, may we embrace the transformative power of emotional intelligence and leverage it to navigate through turbulent times with grace and resilience.

Chapter 9: Building resilience.

———

In the crucible of life's challenges and adversities, resilience emerges as a beacon of hope and strength – a quality that enables us to bounce back from setbacks, overcome obstacles, and thrive amidst the chaos and uncertainty of existence. In this chapter, we delve into the profound significance of resilience, exploring why it is important and offering practical strategies to cultivate this essential quality in our lives.

Why is resilience important?

Resilience is the ability to adapt and thrive in the face of adversity, to bend without breaking, and to emerge from challenges stronger and more empowered than before. It is a quality revered by psychologists, philosophers, and spiritual leaders alike, embodying the indomitable spirit of human potential and growth. While resilience may be tested and forged in the fires of adversity, it is ultimately what enables us to transcend our limitations and realize our full potential.

Firstly, resilience is essential for navigating life's inevitable ups and downs with grace and equanimity. In a world that is fraught with uncertainty and unpredictability, resilience enables us to respond to challenges with resilience and determination, rather than succumbing to despair or hopelessness. By cultivating resilience, we develop the inner strength and fortitude needed to weather the storms of life with courage and resilience.

Moreover, resilience is crucial for maintaining emotional well-being and mental health. In times of stress and adversity, resilient individuals are better able to cope with setbacks and setbacks, maintain a positive outlook on life, and bounce back from difficulties with greater ease. By cultivating resilience, we develop a sense of inner peace and stability that enables us to navigate life's challenges with resilience and grace.

Furthermore, resilience is a key ingredient for achieving long-term success and fulfillment. In a world that prizes achievement and success, resilient individuals are better equipped to persevere through setbacks and setbacks, learn from their mistakes, and persist in the pursuit of their goals and aspirations. By cultivating resilience, we develop the resilience and determination needed to overcome obstacles and achieve our dreams.

Practical strategies to build resilience.

Cultivate a growth mindset: A growth mindset is the belief that our abilities and intelligence can be developed through dedication and hard work. By cultivating a growth mindset, we view challenges as opportunities for growth and learning, rather than insurmountable obstacles. This mindset enables us to approach setbacks with resilience and determination, rather than giving up at the first sign of difficulty.

Develop strong social connections: Social support is a crucial factor in building resilience. By cultivating strong social connections with friends, family, and community members, we create a support network that can help us navigate through life's challenges with resilience and grace. Moreover, spending time with loved ones can provide emotional support, encouragement, and perspective that can help us weather the storms of life more effectively.

Practice self-care: Self-care is essential for maintaining physical, emotional, and mental well-being. By prioritizing activities that nourish and replenish us, such as exercise, meditation, hobbies, and spending time in nature, we cultivate resilience and strength that enables us to cope with stress and adversity more effectively. Moreover, self-care helps us recharge our batteries and replenish our energy reserves, enabling us to face life's challenges with greater resilience and fortitude.

Cultivate mindfulness: Mindfulness is the practice of being fully present in the moment, without judgment or attachment. By cultivating mindfulness through practices such as meditation, deep breathing, or mindful walking, we develop greater awareness of our thoughts, emotions, and reactions. This awareness enables us to respond to challenges with resilience and equanimity, rather than reacting impulsively out of fear or frustration.

Foster optimism and gratitude: Optimism and gratitude are powerful antidotes to stress and adversity. By cultivating an optimistic outlook on life and focusing on the blessings and abundance in our lives, we develop resilience and strength that enables us to navigate through life's challenges with grace and equanimity. Moreover, practicing gratitude can help us shift our perspective from negativity to positivity, enabling us to find silver linings amidst the darkest clouds.

In conclusion, resilience is an essential quality that enables us to navigate life's challenges with grace and fortitude. By cultivating resilience through strategies such as cultivating a growth mindset, developing strong social connections, practicing self-care, cultivating mindfulness, and fostering optimism and gratitude, we develop the inner strength and fortitude needed to overcome obstacles and thrive amidst the chaos and uncertainty of existence. As we embrace the power of resilience, may we cultivate a deeper sense of inner peace and empowerment that enables us to navigate life's challenges with resilience, grace, and dignity.

Chapter 10: Flexibility and adaptability.

———

In the ever-changing landscape of life, flexibility and adaptability stand as essential virtues, guiding us through the shifting tides of uncertainty and change. In this chapter, we explore the profound importance of flexibility in times of change and offer practical insights on how we can improve our adaptability to navigate the complexities of existence.

The importance of flexibility in times of change.

Flexibility is the ability to bend without breaking, to adapt to changing circumstances with grace and resilience. In times of change, flexibility is not merely a luxury but a necessity for survival. It enables us to embrace new challenges, navigate unforeseen obstacles, and thrive amidst uncertainty.

One of the key principles of flexibility is openness to new experiences and perspectives. Instead of clinging rigidly to preconceived notions or expectations, flexible individuals approach life with an open mind and a willingness to embrace the unknown. By cultivating a spirit of curiosity and adventure, we expand our horizons and discover new opportunities for growth and self-discovery.

Moreover, flexibility fosters resilience and emotional well-being. In the face of adversity, flexible individuals are able to adapt to changing circumstances with ease, rather than becoming overwhelmed or discouraged. By maintaining a flexible mindset, we are better equipped to bounce back from setbacks, learn from our experiences, and emerge stronger and more resilient than before.

Furthermore, flexibility promotes innovation and creativity. In a world that is constantly evolving, the ability to adapt to changing circumstances is essential for survival. Flexible individuals are able to think outside the box, explore new possibilities, and find creative solutions to complex problems. By embracing flexibility, we unleash our creative potential and unlock new pathways towards success and fulfillment.

How can we improve our adaptability?

Improving adaptability requires a combination of self-awareness, mindset shifts, and practical strategies. Here are some practical insights on how we can enhance our adaptability to navigate the uncertainties of life:

Cultivate self-awareness: Self-awareness is the foundation of adaptability. By understanding our strengths, weaknesses, and tendencies, we can identify areas where we may need to improve our adaptability. Through practices such as mindfulness, journaling, or self-reflection, we can cultivate greater self-awareness and develop a deeper understanding of ourselves.

Embrace uncertainty: Uncertainty is a natural part of life, and learning to embrace it is essential for building adaptability. Instead of fearing the unknown, we can view uncertainty as an opportunity for growth and exploration. By reframing uncertainty as a catalyst for change and transformation, we can approach new challenges with courage and resilience.

Foster a growth mindset: A growth mindset is the belief that our abilities and intelligence can be developed through effort and perseverance. By adopting a growth mindset, we view challenges as opportunities for learning and growth, rather than obstacles to be avoided. By cultivating a mindset of curiosity and resilience, we can adapt to changing circumstances with ease and confidence.

Practice flexibility: Flexibility is a skill that can be cultivated through practice and repetition. By intentionally exposing ourselves to new experiences, ideas, and perspectives, we can expand our comfort zones and become more adaptable to change. Whether it's trying new activities, learning new skills, or exploring different ways of thinking, practicing flexibility helps us build resilience and adaptability over time.

Build a support network: Building a strong support network of friends, family, and mentors can provide valuable guidance and encouragement during times of change. By surrounding ourselves with supportive and empathetic individuals, we can draw strength from their wisdom and experience, and navigate through uncertainty with greater confidence and resilience.

In conclusion, flexibility and adaptability are essential skills for navigating the complexities of life. By embracing flexibility, cultivating self-awareness, and adopting a growth mindset, we can enhance our adaptability and thrive amidst uncertainty and change. As we continue on our journey of self-discovery and growth, may we embrace the power of flexibility and adaptability to navigate the ever-changing currents of existence with grace and resilience.

Chapter 11: Finding meaning and purpose.

―――

In the labyrinth of existence, amidst the chaos and uncertainty that pervade our lives, lies the eternal quest for meaning and purpose. In this chapter, we delve into the profound importance of finding meaning and purpose, exploring why it is essential for our well-being and resilience, and offering insights on how we can recognize our life's purpose even in the midst of turbulent times.

Why is it important to find meaning and purpose?

Finding meaning and purpose is essential for our overall well-being and fulfillment. It provides us with a sense of direction, motivation, and fulfillment that transcends the transient pleasures and pains of everyday life. Here are some reasons why finding meaning and purpose is important:

Sense of fulfillment: Having a sense of meaning and purpose gives our lives a sense of significance and fulfillment. It allows us to feel that our lives have meaning beyond our individual desires and ambitions, and that our actions have a positive impact on the world around us.

Resilience in the face of adversity: Finding meaning and purpose can provide us with the strength and resilience to withstand life's challenges and setbacks. When we have a clear sense of purpose, we are better able to weather the storms of life with grace and perseverance, knowing that our struggles are part of a larger narrative that gives our lives meaning.

Improved mental and physical health: Research has shown that having a sense of meaning and purpose is correlated with better mental and physical health outcomes. People who report having a strong sense of purpose tend to experience lower levels of stress, anxiety, and depression, and have better overall well-being.

Greater motivation and productivity: When we have a clear sense of purpose, we are more motivated and focused in pursuing our goals and aspirations. Having a sense of meaning can give us the drive and determination to overcome obstacles and persevere in the face of challenges, leading to greater productivity and success.

How can we recognize our life's purpose even in turbulent times?

Recognizing our life's purpose can be challenging, especially in the midst of turbulent times. However, there are several strategies we can employ to uncover our purpose and find meaning in our lives, even in the face of adversity:

Reflect on your values and passions: Take some time to reflect on what matters most to you and what brings you joy and fulfillment. Consider your core values, interests, and passions, and think about how you can align them with your daily activities and goals. Your purpose is likely to be found at the intersection of what you love, what you're good at, and what the world needs.

Pay attention to what energizes you: Notice the activities and experiences that energize and inspire you, even in the midst of challenging times. These moments of flow and engagement can provide valuable clues about your life's purpose and direction. Pay attention to the things that make you feel alive and fulfilled, and consider how you can incorporate more of them into your life.

Seek out opportunities for growth and contribution: Look for opportunities to learn, grow, and make a positive impact in the world around you. Whether it's volunteering, mentoring others, or pursuing personal development goals, finding ways to contribute to something greater than yourself can help you connect with your sense of purpose and meaning.

Embrace uncertainty and change: Recognize that your life's purpose may evolve and change over time, and that's okay. Embrace the uncertainty and unpredictability of life as opportunities for growth and exploration. Stay open to new experiences and possibilities, and trust that your purpose will reveal itself to you in its own time.

Practice self-compassion and patience: Be kind and compassionate with yourself as you navigate the journey of discovering your purpose. Understand that finding meaning and purpose is a lifelong process, and that it's okay to feel uncertain or lost at times. Trust in your own inner wisdom and intuition, and have patience as you explore and uncover your purpose.

In conclusion, finding meaning and purpose is an essential part of the human experience, providing us with a sense of fulfillment, resilience, and direction in life. By reflecting on our values and passions, paying attention to what energizes us, seeking out opportunities for growth and contribution, and embracing uncertainty with self-compassion and patience, we can uncover our life's purpose and find meaning even in the most turbulent times. As we embark on this journey of self-discovery and exploration, may we find solace and inspiration in the knowledge that our lives have meaning and purpose, no matter what challenges we may face along the way.

Chapter 12: Mindfulness and meditation.

———

In the fast-paced and chaotic world we inhabit, the practice of mindfulness and meditation serves as a sanctuary of peace and tranquility amidst the storms of life. In this chapter, we explore the profound role of mindfulness and meditation in stress management, delving into why they are essential practices for promoting well-being and offering practical exercises to cultivate mindfulness and meditation in our daily lives.

The role of mindfulness and meditation in stress management.

Mindfulness and meditation are ancient practices that have been used for centuries to promote physical, mental, and emotional well-being. In recent years, they have gained widespread recognition for their effectiveness in reducing stress, anxiety, and depression, and improving overall quality of life.

One of the key principles of mindfulness and meditation is the cultivation of present-moment awareness. By focusing our attention on the present moment, we become more attuned to our thoughts, emotions, and bodily sensations, and less caught up in worries or regrets about the past or future. This awareness enables us to respond to stressors with greater clarity and equanimity, rather than reacting impulsively out of fear or frustration.

Moreover, mindfulness and meditation promote relaxation and stress reduction by activating the body's natural relaxation response. Through practices such as deep breathing, progressive muscle relaxation, and body scan meditation, we can induce a state of deep relaxation that counteracts the physiological effects of stress and promotes feelings of calm and tranquility.

Furthermore, mindfulness and meditation foster resilience and emotional well-being by cultivating a sense of inner peace and acceptance. By practicing non-judgmental awareness of our thoughts and feelings, we learn to observe them with compassion and detachment, rather than getting caught up in negative thought patterns or self-criticism. This sense of acceptance enables us to navigate through life's challenges with greater resilience and equanimity.

Practical exercises to promote mindfulness and meditation

Mindful breathing: Take a few moments each day to practice mindful breathing. Find a quiet space where you won't be disturbed, and sit or lie down in a comfortable position. Close your eyes and bring your attention to your breath as it enters and leaves your body. Notice the sensation of the breath as it fills your lungs and expands your chest, and then as it leaves your body, releasing tension and stress with each exhale. Continue to focus on your breath for several minutes, allowing yourself to become fully present in the moment.

Body scan meditation: Body scan meditation is a practice that involves systematically scanning your body from head to toe, noticing any sensations or areas of tension or discomfort. Find a comfortable position lying down on your back, with your arms at your sides and your eyes closed. Begin by bringing your attention to your toes, noticing any sensations or tension in this area, and then slowly move your attention upward, scanning each part of your body in turn. Notice any areas of tension or discomfort, and gently breathe into them, allowing them to soften and release.

Loving-kindness meditation: Loving-kindness meditation is a practice that involves sending love and compassion to ourselves and others. Find a comfortable position sitting or lying down, and close your eyes. Begin by bringing to mind someone you love and care about deeply, and silently repeat the following phrases to yourself: "May you be happy, may you be healthy, may you be safe, may you be at peace." Repeat these phrases several times, allowing yourself to feel a sense of love and compassion for this person. Then, gradually expand your circle of compassion to include yourself, and then others in your life, and eventually all beings everywhere.

Mindful walking: Mindful walking is a practice that involves bringing awareness to each step as you walk. Find a quiet place where you can walk without distractions, such as a park or nature trail. Begin by standing still for a moment, and bringing your attention to your feet as they make contact with the ground. Then, slowly begin to walk, noticing the sensation of each foot as it lifts off the ground and then makes contact again. Pay attention to the rhythm of your breath, and the sights, sounds, and smells around you as you walk. Allow yourself to become fully present in the experience of walking, and notice how it feels to be fully engaged in the present moment.

In conclusion, mindfulness and meditation are powerful practices for promoting stress management, relaxation, and emotional well-being. By incorporating these practices into our daily lives through exercises such as mindful breathing, body scan meditation, loving-kindness meditation, and mindful walking, we can cultivate a greater sense of presence, peace, and resilience that enables us to navigate through life's challenges with grace and equanimity. As we continue on our journey of self-discovery and growth, may we embrace the transformative power of mindfulness and meditation to cultivate greater well-being and fulfillment in our lives.

Chapter 13: The power of gratitude.

I n the hustle and bustle of modern life, amidst the chaos and clamor that often surrounds us, lies a simple yet profound practice that has the power to transform our perception of the world – gratitude. In this chapter, we explore the profound importance of gratitude, delving into why it is essential for our well-being and offering insights on how we can cultivate gratitude to find calm amidst the storm.

Why is gratitude important?

Gratitude is more than just a fleeting feeling of thankfulness; it is a transformative mindset and way of life that can profoundly impact our well-being and outlook on life. Here are some reasons why gratitude is important:

Shifts our perspective: Gratitude has the power to shift our perspective from scarcity to abundance, from focusing on what we lack to appreciating what we have. By cultivating a mindset of gratitude, we train ourselves to see the blessings and beauty that surround us, even amidst difficult circumstances.

Fosters resilience: Gratitude is a powerful tool for building resilience in the face of adversity. When we practice gratitude, we train our minds to focus on the positive aspects of our lives, rather than dwelling on the negative. This positive outlook helps us navigate through challenges with greater grace and resilience, knowing that there is always something to be grateful for, even in the darkest of times.

Improves mental and physical health: Research has shown that practicing gratitude is correlated with numerous health benefits, including improved mood, reduced stress levels, and better overall well-being. Grateful individuals tend to experience lower levels of anxiety and depression, better sleep quality, and enhanced immune function.

Strengthens relationships: Gratitude has the power to deepen our connections with others and foster a sense of belonging and community. When we express gratitude towards others, we strengthen our bonds with them and create a positive feedback loop of kindness and appreciation. This, in turn, enhances our own sense of happiness and fulfillment.

How can we practice gratitude to find calm?

Practicing gratitude is a simple yet powerful way to cultivate a sense of calm and contentment in our lives, even amidst the chaos and uncertainty that surrounds us. Here are some practical strategies to help you incorporate gratitude into your daily routine:

Keep a gratitude journal: Start a gratitude journal where you can write down three things you are grateful for each day. They can be big or small, simple or profound – the key is to focus on the blessings and abundance in your life rather than dwelling on what is lacking. Taking a few moments each day to reflect on the things you are grateful for can shift your perspective and bring a sense of peace and contentment.

Practice mindfulness: Incorporate mindfulness practices into your daily routine, such as mindful breathing, meditation, or mindful walking. Mindfulness helps us cultivate awareness of the present moment and appreciate the beauty and richness of life. By being fully present and attentive to the present moment, we can more easily recognize and savor the things we are grateful for.

Express gratitude to others: Take the time to express gratitude to the people in your life who have made a positive impact on you. Write a thank-you note, send a text or email expressing your appreciation, or simply say "thank you" in person. By acknowledging and expressing gratitude towards others, we strengthen our relationships and create a sense of connection and belonging.

Count your blessings: Take a moment each day to mentally count your blessings and acknowledge the things you are grateful for. Whether it's your health, your loved ones, or the beauty of nature, take the time to appreciate the abundance and richness of your life. By focusing on the positive aspects of your life, you can cultivate a sense of calm and contentment that transcends external circumstances.

Practice gratitude rituals: Incorporate gratitude rituals into your daily routine, such as saying a prayer of thanks before meals, keeping a gratitude jar where you can write down things you are grateful for throughout the day, or setting aside time each evening to reflect on the things you are thankful for. These simple rituals can help you cultivate a mindset of gratitude and bring a sense of peace and joy to your life.

In conclusion, gratitude is a powerful practice that has the power to transform our lives and bring a sense of calm and contentment amidst the chaos of modern life. By cultivating a mindset of gratitude and incorporating simple practices into our daily routine, we can enhance our well-being, strengthen our relationships, and find peace and fulfillment in the present moment. As we embark on this journey of gratitude and self-discovery, may we embrace the power of gratitude to cultivate a deeper sense of calm and contentment in our lives.

Chapter 14: Supportive relationships.

———

In the intricate tapestry of human existence, supportive relationships serve as the sturdy threads that weave together moments of joy, comfort, and resilience. In this chapter, we explore the profound importance of supportive relationships in difficult times, and offer insights on how we can strengthen our connections with others to find calm amidst life's storms.

The importance of supportive relationships in difficult times.

Supportive relationships are essential for our emotional well-being and resilience, providing us with a sense of belonging, acceptance, and security. In times of difficulty and uncertainty, supportive relationships serve as a source of strength and solace, offering us comfort, guidance, and reassurance when we need it most.

Firstly, supportive relationships provide us with a sense of belonging and connection. When we feel connected to others, we experience a sense of belonging and acceptance that nourishes our soul and fosters a sense of security and well-being. Knowing that we have a network of people who care about us and support us unconditionally can provide us with the courage and resilience to face life's challenges with grace and confidence.

Moreover, supportive relationships offer us emotional support and validation. In times of crisis or distress, having someone to talk to and share our feelings with can be incredibly comforting and healing. Supportive friends, family members, or mentors can provide us with a listening ear, a shoulder to lean on, and words of encouragement that help us navigate through difficult times with greater ease and resilience.

Furthermore, supportive relationships offer us practical assistance and guidance. Whether it's helping us brainstorm solutions to a problem, offering us practical advice, or simply lending a helping hand, supportive relationships can provide us with the resources and support we need to overcome obstacles and move forward in life.

How can we strengthen our relationships to find calm?

Strengthening our relationships requires intention, effort, and a willingness to cultivate empathy, compassion, and understanding. Here are some practical insights on how we can strengthen our relationships to find calm amidst life's challenges:

Practice active listening: One of the most powerful ways to strengthen relationships is through active listening. When we truly listen to others with empathy and compassion, we validate their experiences and feelings, and create a deeper sense of connection and understanding. Practice active listening by giving your full attention to the speaker, maintaining eye contact, and offering validating responses that show you understand and empathize with their perspective.

Express gratitude and appreciation: Gratitude is a powerful tool for strengthening relationships and fostering a sense of connection and appreciation. Take the time to express gratitude and appreciation to the people in your life who support and uplift you. Whether it's a heartfelt thank-you note, a small gesture of kindness, or simply expressing your appreciation in words, expressing gratitude can deepen your relationships and foster a sense of mutual respect and appreciation.

Foster empathy and compassion: Empathy and compassion are essential qualities for building strong and supportive relationships. Practice empathy by putting yourself in the other person's shoes and trying to understand their perspective and feelings. Show compassion by offering support, encouragement, and understanding to those who are going through difficult times. By fostering empathy and compassion in your relationships, you create a safe and supportive environment where people feel understood, valued, and accepted.

Set healthy boundaries: Setting healthy boundaries is essential for maintaining healthy and fulfilling relationships. Boundaries help us establish clear expectations and guidelines for how we want to be treated and how we will treat others. By setting and respecting boundaries in our relationships, we create a sense of safety and trust that allows us to be authentic and vulnerable with each other.

Make time for connection: In our fast-paced and busy world, it's easy to neglect our relationships and prioritize other commitments. However, making time for connection is essential for strengthening relationships and fostering a sense of intimacy and closeness. Set aside dedicated time each week to spend quality time with the people you care about, whether it's having a meaningful conversation over coffee, going for a walk together, or simply enjoying each other's company.

In conclusion, supportive relationships are essential for our emotional well-being and resilience, providing us with a sense of belonging, acceptance, and security. By actively listening, expressing gratitude and appreciation, fostering empathy and compassion, setting healthy boundaries, and making time for connection, we can strengthen our relationships and find calm amidst life's storms. As we nurture our connections with others, may we find solace and strength in the knowledge that we are not alone, and that we have a network of supportive relationships to lean on in times of need.

Chapter 15: Time management in turbulent times.

―――

In the whirlwind of modern life, where chaos and demands constantly vie for our attention, effective time management stands as a beacon of order and control. In this chapter, we explore the significance of time management in turbulent times, offering practical tips and strategies to help us better organize our time and find calm amidst the storm.

The importance of time management.

Time is perhaps the most precious resource we possess, yet it is finite and irreplaceable. In turbulent times, when demands on our time and attention seem to multiply exponentially, effective time management becomes essential for maintaining balance, productivity, and well-being.

Minimize distractions: In today's hyper-connected world, distractions abound at every turn, making it challenging to stay focused and productive. To better manage your time, identify and minimize distractions that sap your energy and productivity. This may involve turning off notifications on your phone, setting boundaries with colleagues or family members, or creating a dedicated workspace free from distractions.

Prioritize tasks: Not all tasks are created equal, and prioritizing is key to effective time management. Take some time at the beginning of each day to identify your most important tasks and prioritize them based on their urgency and importance. This will help you focus your time and energy on the tasks that will have the greatest impact on your goals and objectives.

Break tasks into smaller steps: Large, daunting tasks can be overwhelming and lead to procrastination. To make them more manageable, break them down into smaller, more manageable steps.

This will help you make progress on your tasks incrementally and prevent feelings of overwhelm or paralysis.

Set deadlines and goals: Deadlines and goals provide structure and motivation to your work, helping you stay focused and on track. Set realistic deadlines for your tasks and projects, and break them down into smaller milestones to track your progress. Celebrate your achievements along the way, and adjust your goals and deadlines as needed to stay aligned with your priorities.

Learn to say no: In turbulent times, it's easy to become overwhelmed by commitments and obligations. Learning to say no to non-essential tasks or requests can help you better manage your time and protect your energy. Prioritize your own well-being and focus on the tasks that align with your goals and priorities.

Delegate tasks: You don't have to do everything yourself. Delegating tasks to others can help you free up time and focus on your highest priorities. Identify tasks that can be delegated to colleagues, family members, or outsourcing services, and empower others to take on responsibilities and contribute to the success of your projects.

Take breaks and recharge: In the midst of a busy schedule, it's important to take regular breaks to rest and recharge. Schedule short breaks throughout your day to step away from your work, stretch, and clear your mind. This will help you maintain focus and productivity over the long term and prevent burnout.

Practice self-care: Self-care is essential for maintaining your physical, emotional, and mental well-being, especially in turbulent times. Make time for activities that nourish your body, mind, and soul, such as exercise, meditation, hobbies, and spending time with loved ones. By prioritizing self-care, you'll have more energy and resilience to tackle the challenges of daily life.

In conclusion, effective time management is essential for finding calm and maintaining balance in turbulent times. By minimizing distractions, prioritizing tasks, setting deadlines and goals, learning to say no, delegating tasks, taking breaks and recharging, and practicing self-care, you can better organize your time and focus your energy on the tasks that matter most. As you implement these strategies into your daily routine, may you find greater clarity, productivity, and well-being, even amidst the chaos and demands of modern life.

Chapter 16: Setting boundaries.

———

In the tumultuous sea of life, setting boundaries acts as a sturdy vessel, guiding us through choppy waters and ensuring our well-being amidst the storm. In this chapter, we explore the significance of boundaries in stressful situations, understanding why they are crucial for our mental and emotional health, and offer insights into how we can learn to set healthy boundaries.

The importance of boundaries in stressful situations.

Boundaries serve as the invisible lines that delineate our personal space, values, and limits. In stressful situations, boundaries play a pivotal role in protecting our physical, emotional, and mental well-being. Here's why boundaries are crucial:

Preserving self-respect: Boundaries help us maintain a sense of self-respect and dignity by defining what is acceptable and unacceptable behavior from others. They prevent us from being taken advantage of or mistreated and empower us to assert our needs and values.

Protecting mental and emotional health: Stressful situations can take a toll on our mental and emotional health, leading to burnout, anxiety, and depression. Boundaries act as a shield, protecting us from toxic relationships, excessive demands, and emotional manipulation. They help us create space for self-care, rest, and relaxation, essential for maintaining our well-being.

Promoting healthy relationships: Boundaries are essential for fostering healthy, mutually respectful relationships. They allow us to communicate our needs and expectations clearly, establish trust and respect, and navigate conflicts and disagreements constructively. By setting and respecting boundaries, we create a foundation of trust and safety that strengthens our connections with others.

Enhancing productivity and focus: Boundaries help us maintain focus and productivity by minimizing distractions and interruptions. They enable us to create a conducive environment for work, study, or creative pursuits, free from unnecessary noise, interruptions, or intrusions. By setting boundaries around our time and space, we can optimize our productivity and achieve our goals more efficiently.

How can we learn to set healthy boundaries?

Learning to set healthy boundaries is a skill that requires self-awareness, assertiveness, and practice. Here are some insights into how we can cultivate this skill:

Know your values and limits: Reflect on your values, needs, and limits to identify what is important to you and where you draw the line. Be clear about your priorities, preferences, and non-negotiables, and communicate them assertively to others.

Communicate assertively: Assertive communication is key to setting and enforcing boundaries effectively. Clearly and respectfully communicate your boundaries to others, using "I" statements to express your needs and expectations. Be firm and confident in asserting your boundaries, and don't be afraid to say no when necessary.

Practice self-care: Prioritize self-care and make time for activities that nourish your body, mind, and soul. Setting boundaries around your time and energy is essential for protecting your well-being and preventing burnout. Learn to say no to activities or commitments that drain your energy or detract from your well-being.

Set boundaries with compassion: Setting boundaries doesn't mean shutting others out or being hostile. Approach boundary-setting with compassion and empathy, understanding that boundaries are essential for maintaining healthy relationships and self-respect.

Communicate your boundaries with kindness and understanding, and be willing to listen to others' perspectives.

Be consistent and firm: Consistency is key to maintaining boundaries over time. Once you've established your boundaries, stick to them consistently, even when it's challenging. Be firm in enforcing your boundaries and don't allow others to push past them or disregard your needs.

Seek support if needed: If you're struggling to set or enforce boundaries, don't hesitate to seek support from trusted friends, family members, or a therapist. They can offer guidance, encouragement, and practical strategies to help you establish and maintain healthy boundaries in your life.

In conclusion, setting boundaries is essential for protecting our well-being and fostering healthy relationships, especially in stressful situations. By knowing our values and limits, communicating assertively, practicing self-care, setting boundaries with compassion, being consistent and firm, and seeking support when needed, we can learn to set healthy boundaries that promote our mental, emotional, and physical health. As we cultivate this skill, may we find greater peace, balance, and resilience in navigating life's challenges and uncertainties.

Chapter 17: Creativity as an outlet.

———

In the tumultuous storms of life, creativity stands as a beacon of light, offering solace and sanctuary amidst chaos and uncertainty. In this chapter, we explore the profound role of creativity as an outlet for coping with chaos, and we uncover ways in which we can harness our creative abilities to find calm and inspiration in the midst of life's challenges.

The role of creativity in coping with chaos.

Creativity is more than just a talent or skill; it is a fundamental aspect of human nature that allows us to express ourselves, explore new possibilities, and make sense of the world around us. In times of chaos and upheaval, creativity serves as a powerful outlet for processing emotions, finding meaning, and fostering resilience.

Expressing emotions: In times of stress and uncertainty, emotions can run high, leaving us feeling overwhelmed and vulnerable. Creativity provides a safe and healthy outlet for expressing and processing these emotions, allowing us to channel our thoughts and feelings into creative endeavors such as writing, painting, music, or dance. Through creative expression, we can release pent-up emotions, gain insight into our innermost thoughts and feelings, and find catharsis and healing.

Finding meaning: Chaos often disrupts our sense of meaning and purpose, leaving us feeling adrift and disoriented. Creativity offers a pathway towards finding meaning amidst the chaos, as it allows us to explore our values, beliefs, and aspirations through creative expression. Whether through storytelling, visual art, or music, creativity enables us to make sense of our experiences, find connection and resonance with others, and discover deeper truths about ourselves and the world around us.

Fostering resilience: Creativity fosters resilience by providing us with a sense of agency and empowerment in the face of adversity. When we engage in creative activities, we tap into our innate ability to adapt, innovate, and problem-solve, which strengthens our ability to navigate challenges and overcome obstacles. Creativity encourages us to embrace experimentation and risk-taking, to think outside the box, and to approach problems with curiosity and flexibility, all of which are essential qualities for building resilience in turbulent times.

How can we use our creativity to find calm?

Engage in creative activities: Take time each day to engage in creative activities that bring you joy and inspiration. Whether it's painting, writing, cooking, gardening, or playing a musical instrument, find activities that allow you to express yourself and tap into your creative flow. Set aside dedicated time for creative pursuits, and allow yourself to immerse fully in the process without judgment or expectation.

Practice mindful creativity: Approach your creative endeavors with a spirit of mindfulness and presence, allowing yourself to fully immerse in the creative process. Pay attention to the sensations, thoughts, and emotions that arise as you engage in creative activities, and allow them to inform and inspire your work. Cultivate a sense of curiosity and openness, and trust in your intuition and inner wisdom as you explore new ideas and possibilities.

Embrace imperfection: Let go of perfectionism and embrace the beauty of imperfection in your creative endeavors. Allow yourself to make mistakes, take risks, and experiment with new techniques and ideas. Remember that creativity is a journey of exploration and discovery, and that each mistake or misstep is an opportunity for growth and learning. Celebrate your progress and accomplishments along the way, and be gentle and compassionate with yourself as you navigate the creative process.

Find inspiration in nature: Nature is a boundless source of inspiration and creativity, offering endless opportunities for exploration and discovery. Spend time outdoors, soaking in the sights, sounds, and sensations of the natural world, and allow yourself to be inspired by its beauty and majesty. Take walks in the park, hike in the mountains, or simply sit in your backyard and observe the world around you. Allow nature to nourish your soul and ignite your creative spark.

In conclusion, creativity serves as a powerful outlet for coping with chaos, offering solace, inspiration, and resilience in times of uncertainty and upheaval. By engaging in creative activities, practicing mindful creativity, embracing imperfection, and finding inspiration in nature, we can tap into our innate creative potential and harness it as a tool for finding calm and meaning amidst the chaos of life. As we embrace our creativity and allow it to guide us on our journey of self-discovery and growth, may we find solace and inspiration in the beauty and wonder of the creative process.

Chapter 18: Seeking harmony.

———

In the cacophony of life's challenges and uncertainties, the pursuit of harmony stands as a beacon of hope and resilience. In this chapter, we explore the profound significance of harmony and its role in fostering well-being and balance amidst chaos. We'll delve into why harmony is important and offer insights on how we can cultivate it amidst life's turbulence.

Why is harmony important?

Harmony is more than just a pleasant arrangement of sounds or colors; it is a state of balance, alignment, and integration that brings a sense of peace and coherence to our lives. Here are some reasons why harmony is important:

Inner peace: Harmony cultivates a sense of inner peace and tranquility by aligning our thoughts, emotions, and actions with our values and aspirations. When we are in harmony with ourselves, we experience a deep sense of contentment and well-being that transcends the ups and downs of external circumstances.

Health and well-being: Research has shown that harmony is closely linked to physical and mental health. When our body, mind, and spirit are in harmony, we experience greater resilience to stress, reduced levels of anxiety and depression, and improved overall well-being. Cultivating harmony in our lives promotes a state of balance and vitality that supports our health and vitality.

Relationships: Harmony fosters harmonious relationships with others by promoting empathy, understanding, and cooperation. When we are in harmony with others, we experience deeper connections and more meaningful interactions, leading to greater intimacy, trust, and mutual support.

Creativity and productivity: Harmony stimulates creativity and productivity by creating an environment conducive to innovation and collaboration. When we are in harmony with our environment and our inner selves, we are better able to tap into our creative potential, solve problems creatively, and achieve our goals with greater efficiency and effectiveness.

How can we find harmony amidst chaos?

Cultivate self-awareness: Begin by cultivating self-awareness and introspection to understand your values, priorities, and innermost desires. Take time to reflect on what brings you joy and fulfillment, and identify areas of your life where you may be out of alignment with your true self. By aligning your thoughts, emotions, and actions with your core values, you can cultivate a greater sense of harmony and authenticity in your life.

Practice mindfulness: Mindfulness is the practice of being fully present in the moment, without judgment or attachment. By cultivating mindfulness through meditation, deep breathing, or mindful awareness, you can become more attuned to the rhythms and patterns of your life, and more able to respond to challenges with grace and equanimity. Mindfulness helps you cultivate a sense of inner peace and harmony amidst the chaos and turmoil of daily life.

Seek balance: Strive to find balance in all areas of your life, including work, relationships, and personal well-being. Identify areas where you may be overextending yourself or neglecting your needs, and take steps to restore balance and harmony. This may involve setting boundaries, prioritizing self-care, or reallocating your time and energy to align with your values and priorities.

Cultivate gratitude: Gratitude is the practice of appreciating the blessings and abundance in your life, even amidst challenges and difficulties. By cultivating gratitude through practices such as keeping a gratitude journal or expressing appreciation to others, you can shift your focus from what is lacking to what is abundant and meaningful in your life. Gratitude fosters a sense of harmony and contentment that transcends external circumstances.

Embrace change: Embrace change as a natural part of life's ebb and flow, and approach it with an open mind and heart. Instead of resisting change or clinging to the familiar, embrace the opportunities for growth and transformation that change brings. Trust in the process of life and allow yourself to flow with the currents of change, knowing that harmony arises from embracing the natural rhythms of existence.

In conclusion, seeking harmony amidst chaos is a journey of self-discovery and self-realization that requires patience, practice, and perseverance. By cultivating self-awareness, practicing mindfulness, seeking balance, cultivating gratitude, and embracing change, you can cultivate a greater sense of harmony and well-being in your life. As you embark on this journey, may you find solace and inspiration in the beauty and wonder of life's ever-unfolding dance, and may you discover the harmony that resides within your own heart and soul.

Chapter 19: The art of saying no.

———

In a world filled with endless demands and obligations, mastering the art of saying no is a crucial skill for preserving our time, energy, and well-being. In this chapter, we delve into the importance of saying no and provide insights on how to do so appropriately, empowering you to set boundaries and prioritize your needs in a way that fosters balance and harmony in your life.

Why is it important to say no?

Saying no is more than just declining a request or invitation; it is an assertion of our boundaries, priorities, and values. Here are several reasons why saying no is important:

> Preserves time and energy: Our time and energy are finite resources, and saying no allows us to allocate them in alignment with our priorities and goals. By declining requests or commitments that do not serve our best interests, we free up valuable time and energy to invest in activities that nourish and fulfill us.

> Protects boundaries: Saying no is essential for establishing and maintaining healthy boundaries in our relationships and interactions with others. It communicates to others that our needs and well-being are important and deserve respect, and it helps prevent burnout and resentment from overcommitting ourselves.

> Promotes self-care: Saying no is an act of self-care, allowing us to prioritize our own needs and well-being without guilt or apology. It enables us to set aside time for rest, relaxation, and activities that rejuvenate and replenish us, fostering greater resilience and vitality in the face of life's challenges.

> Supports authenticity: Saying no authentically reflects our values, priorities, and personal boundaries. It enables us to live in alignment

with our true selves, rather than conforming to the expectations or demands of others. By honoring our own needs and desires, we cultivate a greater sense of authenticity and integrity in our lives.

How can we learn to say no appropriately?

Learning to say no appropriately requires practice, self-awareness, and assertiveness. Here are some strategies for mastering the art of saying no:

Know your priorities: Take time to clarify your priorities and values, so you can make informed decisions about how to allocate your time and energy. Identify the activities, commitments, and relationships that are most important to you, and use them as a guide for determining when to say no.

Set boundaries: Establish clear boundaries around your time, energy, and resources, and communicate them assertively to others. Be firm but respectful in asserting your boundaries, and be willing to enforce them when necessary. Remember that saying no is not a rejection of others but a protection of yourself.

Practice assertiveness: Assertiveness is the ability to express your needs, opinions, and boundaries in a clear and respectful manner. Practice assertive communication techniques, such as using "I" statements, maintaining eye contact, and speaking confidently and calmly. Be direct and concise in your response, and avoid over-explaining or apologizing for your decision.

Offer alternatives: If you're unable to say yes to a request, offer alternatives or compromises that may meet the other person's needs while still respecting your own boundaries. For example, you could suggest a different time or date for a meeting, or recommend someone else who may be better suited to help.

Practice self-compassion: Be kind and compassionate with yourself as you learn to say no. Recognize that it's okay to prioritize your own needs and well-being, and that saying no is an act of self-care, not selfishness. Give yourself permission to decline requests without guilt or shame, and trust that you are making the best decision for yourself in that moment.

In conclusion, mastering the art of saying no is an essential skill for preserving our time, energy, and well-being in a world filled with endless demands and obligations. By clarifying our priorities, setting boundaries, practicing assertiveness, offering alternatives, and practicing self-compassion, we can learn to say no appropriately and assertively, empowering us to live with greater authenticity, balance, and harmony in our lives. As we embrace the power of no, may we reclaim our time and energy for the activities and relationships that truly matter to us, and may we cultivate a greater sense of peace and fulfillment in the process.

Chapter 20: The importance of self-care.

———

In the midst of life's chaos and turbulence, self-care emerges as a beacon of solace and resilience, offering a pathway to nurture our physical, emotional, and mental well-being. In this chapter, we explore the profound importance of self-care and provide practical techniques to cultivate self-care in turbulent times, empowering you to prioritize your health and happiness amidst life's challenges.

Why is self-care crucial?

Self-care is the practice of deliberately tending to one's own physical, emotional, and mental needs in order to maintain overall well-being and prevent burnout. Here are several reasons why self-care is crucial:

Enhances resilience: Self-care builds resilience by replenishing our physical, emotional, and mental resources, enabling us to cope more effectively with stress and adversity. By prioritizing self-care, we strengthen our capacity to bounce back from setbacks and challenges, and to face life's difficulties with greater equanimity and grace.

Promotes health and well-being: Self-care is essential for maintaining our physical health and vitality. It involves activities such as regular exercise, nutritious eating, adequate sleep, and preventive healthcare measures, all of which contribute to our overall health and longevity. By prioritizing self-care, we reduce the risk of illness and disease, and promote optimal functioning of our bodies and minds.

Fosters emotional balance: Self-care supports emotional well-being by providing opportunities for relaxation, self-reflection, and emotional expression. Activities such as journaling, meditation, mindfulness, and spending time in nature help us regulate our emotions, reduce stress, and cultivate a greater sense of inner peace and serenity.

Strengthens relationships: Self-care enhances our ability to nurture healthy relationships with others by ensuring that we are able to show up fully present and engaged in our interactions. When we take care of ourselves, we are better able to offer support, empathy, and compassion to others, and to maintain healthy boundaries in our relationships.

Practical self-care techniques for turbulent times.

Establish a self-care routine: Create a daily self-care routine that includes activities to nourish your body, mind, and spirit. This may include exercise, meditation, journaling, reading, or engaging in hobbies and activities that bring you joy and fulfillment. Set aside dedicated time each day for self-care, and prioritize it as you would any other important task.

Practice mindfulness: Mindfulness is the practice of being fully present in the moment, without judgment or attachment. Incorporate mindfulness into your daily routine through practices such as meditation, deep breathing, or mindful walking. These practices help you cultivate greater awareness of your thoughts, emotions, and sensations, and promote a sense of calm and inner peace.

Prioritize sleep: Adequate sleep is essential for physical, emotional, and mental well-being. Prioritize sleep by establishing a regular sleep schedule, creating a restful sleep environment, and practicing relaxation techniques before bedtime. Aim for 7-9 hours of quality sleep each night to support optimal health and functioning.

Nourish your body: Pay attention to your nutritional needs and fuel your body with wholesome, nourishing foods. Eat a balanced diet rich in fruits, vegetables, whole grains, and lean proteins, and limit consumption of processed foods, sugary snacks, and caffeine. Stay hydrated by drinking plenty of water throughout the day, and listen to your body's hunger and fullness cues.

Engage in physical activity: Regular physical activity is essential for maintaining physical health and reducing stress. Find activities that you enjoy and make them a regular part of your routine, whether it's going for a walk, practicing yoga, or participating in a group fitness class. Aim for at least 30 minutes of moderate-intensity exercise most days of the week to support overall health and well-being.

Cultivate supportive relationships: Surround yourself with supportive friends, family members, and community members who uplift and inspire you. Reach out to others for support when needed, and offer support and encouragement to those in your network. Cultivating strong social connections is essential for emotional well-being and resilience in turbulent times.

Practice self-compassion: Be kind and compassionate with yourself as you navigate the ups and downs of life. Treat yourself with the same kindness and understanding that you would offer to a close friend, and practice self-compassion in moments of difficulty or self-doubt. Remember that self-care is not selfish, but essential for maintaining your health and well-being.

In conclusion, self-care is a crucial practice for nurturing our physical, emotional, and mental well-being amidst life's turbulence. By prioritizing self-care and incorporating practical techniques into our daily lives, we can cultivate resilience, promote health and well-being, and find greater peace and fulfillment amidst life's challenges. As we embrace self-care as a priority, may we honor our needs and nurture our souls, fostering a deeper sense of balance, vitality, and joy in our lives.

Chapter 21: Dealing with uncertainty.

———

In the tapestry of life, uncertainty weaves its intricate threads, casting shadows of doubt and fear upon our path. Yet, amidst the chaos and confusion, lies an opportunity for growth, resilience, and transformation. In this chapter, we delve into the profound challenge of coping with uncertainty, exploring strategies to navigate its tumultuous waters with courage and grace.

How can we learn to cope with uncertainty?

Cultivate acceptance: The first step in coping with uncertainty is to cultivate acceptance of the reality that uncertainty is an inherent part of life. Rather than resisting or denying uncertainty, acknowledge it with compassion and openness. Acceptance allows us to release the need for control and surrender to the flow of life, trusting that we have the inner resources to navigate whatever challenges may arise.

Practice mindfulness: Mindfulness is a powerful tool for coping with uncertainty, as it helps us stay grounded in the present moment and cultivate inner peace amidst external turmoil. By practicing mindfulness meditation, deep breathing, or mindful awareness, we can develop greater resilience and equanimity in the face of uncertainty. Mindfulness allows us to observe our thoughts and emotions without judgment, and to respond to challenges with clarity and composure.

Cultivate resilience: Resilience is the ability to bounce back from adversity and grow stronger in the process. Cultivating resilience involves developing coping skills, such as problem-solving, emotion regulation, and social support. By building resilience, we can better adapt to the uncertainties of life and navigate challenges with confidence and grace.

Focus on what you can control: While there are many things in life that are beyond our control, there are also aspects of our lives that we can influence and shape. Focus your energy on what you can control, such as your thoughts, actions, and attitudes. By taking proactive steps to address challenges and pursue your goals, you can regain a sense of agency and empowerment in the face of uncertainty.

Practice self-compassion: Uncertainty can trigger feelings of fear, anxiety, and self-doubt. Practice self-compassion by treating yourself with kindness and understanding during times of uncertainty. Be gentle with yourself as you navigate the unknown, and remind yourself that it's okay to feel uncertain or scared. Self-compassion helps us cultivate resilience and inner strength, enabling us to weather life's storms with greater ease and grace.

Strategies for dealing with fear and uncertainty

Identify your fears: Start by identifying the specific fears and anxieties that are arising in response to uncertainty. Name your fears and acknowledge them with compassion and curiosity. Understanding the root causes of your fears can help you develop strategies for coping with them more effectively.

Challenge negative thoughts: Fear and uncertainty often give rise to negative thoughts and beliefs that can exacerbate our anxiety and stress. Challenge these negative thoughts by questioning their validity and reframing them in a more positive and realistic light. Replace catastrophic thinking with more balanced and rational perspectives, and focus on evidence-based reasoning rather than speculation.

Practice relaxation techniques: Engage in relaxation techniques such as deep breathing, progressive muscle relaxation, or guided imagery to help calm your mind and body during times of uncertainty. These techniques can help reduce feelings of anxiety and promote a sense of calm and relaxation.

Stay connected: Reach out to friends, family members, or support groups for emotional support and reassurance during times of uncertainty. Sharing your fears and concerns with others can help alleviate feelings of isolation and provide validation and encouragement. Strengthening your social connections can also help you feel more supported and resilient in the face of uncertainty.

Focus on the present moment: Instead of dwelling on worst-case scenarios or worrying about the future, focus on the present moment and what you can do to take care of yourself in the here and now. Practice mindfulness and engage in activities that bring you joy and fulfillment, such as spending time in nature, practicing a hobby, or connecting with loved ones.

In conclusion, coping with uncertainty is a challenging but essential aspect of the human experience. By cultivating acceptance, practicing mindfulness, building resilience, focusing on what you can control, and practicing self-compassion, you can navigate uncertainty with courage and grace. Remember that uncertainty is a natural part of life, and that you have the inner resources and resilience to cope with whatever challenges may arise. As you cultivate these strategies for dealing with fear and uncertainty, may you find greater peace, resilience, and inner strength to navigate life's uncertainties with courage and grace.

Chapter 22: The power of positivity.

———

In the intricate tapestry of life, positivity shines as a radiant thread, weaving resilience, hope, and fulfillment into the fabric of our existence. In this chapter, we explore the transformative effects of positive thinking on our resilience and well-being. We'll delve into the profound impact of cultivating a positive attitude and offer practical insights on how to foster positivity in our lives, even amidst the most challenging circumstances.

The effects of positive thinking on our resilience.

Positive thinking is not merely a state of mind; it is a powerful force that shapes our perception of the world and influences our actions and outcomes. Here are several ways in which cultivating a positive attitude can enhance our resilience and well-being:

Resilience in the face of adversity: Positive thinking enables us to approach challenges and setbacks with optimism and resilience. Instead of viewing obstacles as insurmountable barriers, we see them as opportunities for growth and learning. By reframing negative experiences in a more positive light, we can bounce back from adversity with greater strength and determination.

Enhanced mental and emotional well-being: Positive thinking has been linked to improved mental and emotional well-being, including lower levels of stress, anxiety, and depression. When we focus on the positive aspects of our lives and cultivate an attitude of gratitude and optimism, we experience greater happiness, contentment, and inner peace.

Improved physical health: Research has shown that positive thinking can have a positive impact on our physical health, including lower blood pressure, reduced risk of cardiovascular disease, and enhanced immune function. By reducing stress and promoting relaxation, positivity supports our body's natural healing mechanisms and strengthens our overall health and vitality.

Greater success and achievement: Positive thinking is associated with greater success and achievement in both personal and professional domains. When we approach tasks and goals with a positive mindset, we are more likely to persevere in the face of challenges, take initiative, and seize opportunities for growth and advancement.

How can we cultivate a positive attitude?

Practice gratitude: Gratitude is the practice of acknowledging and appreciating the blessings and abundance in our lives, even amidst challenges and difficulties. Cultivate gratitude by keeping a gratitude journal, expressing appreciation to others, or simply taking time each day to reflect on the things you are thankful for. By focusing on the positive aspects of your life, you can cultivate a more positive outlook and enhance your resilience and well-being.

Challenge negative Thoughts: Pay attention to negative thoughts and beliefs that may be holding you back, and challenge them with more positive and empowering alternatives. Instead of dwelling on what could go wrong, focus on what could go right. Practice reframing negative experiences in a more positive light, and adopt a growth mindset that embraces challenges as opportunities for learning and growth.

Surround yourself with positivity: Surround yourself with positive influences, including supportive friends, inspiring role models, and uplifting media. Limit exposure to negative news and social media, and seek out sources of inspiration and encouragement that uplift and energize you. Cultivate a positive environment that fosters optimism and resilience.

Practice self-compassion: Be kind and compassionate with yourself, especially during times of difficulty or struggle. Treat yourself with the same kindness and understanding that you would offer to a friend in need. Practice self-care activities that nourish and replenish your body, mind, and spirit, and give yourself permission to rest and recharge when needed.

Set positive goals: Set goals that align with your values and aspirations, and approach them with a positive attitude and belief in your ability to succeed. Break goals down into manageable steps, and celebrate your progress and achievements along the way. Visualize yourself achieving your goals and experiencing the positive outcomes that result from your efforts.

In conclusion, the power of positivity is a force for transformation and resilience in our lives. By cultivating a positive attitude through practices such as gratitude, challenging negative thoughts, surrounding ourselves with positivity, practicing self-compassion, and setting positive goals, we can enhance our resilience, well-being, and success. As we harness the power of positivity to navigate life's challenges and uncertainties, may we discover the boundless potential for growth, fulfillment, and joy that resides within each of us.

Chapter 23: The role of humor.

———

Humor, with its whimsical charm and infectious joy, serves as a beacon of light in the darkest of times, offering solace, perspective, and resilience amidst life's challenges. In this chapter, we explore the profound role of humor in our lives, examining why it is important and how we can harness its power to cope with adversity and find moments of levity and laughter, even amidst the most trying circumstances.

Why is humor important?

Humor is not merely a source of entertainment; it is a fundamental aspect of the human experience that enriches our lives in myriad ways. Here are several reasons why humor is important:

Stress relief: Humor has a remarkable ability to alleviate stress and tension, providing a much-needed respite from the pressures and demands of daily life. Laughter triggers the release of endorphins, the body's natural feel-good chemicals, which promote relaxation and reduce the physical symptoms of stress.

Emotional resilience: Humor fosters emotional resilience by helping us maintain a lighthearted perspective on life's challenges and setbacks. By finding humor in difficult situations, we can reframe negative experiences in a more positive light and bounce back from adversity with greater ease and grace.

Social connection: Humor strengthens social bonds and fosters a sense of connection and camaraderie with others. Shared laughter creates a sense of unity and belonging, breaking down barriers and fostering empathy, understanding, and mutual support.

Cognitive flexibility: Humor stimulates cognitive flexibility and creativity, encouraging us to think outside the box and approach problems from new perspectives. By challenging our preconceived notions and expanding our mental horizons, humor enhances our problem-solving skills and fosters innovation and adaptability.

How can we use humor to cope with challenges?

Find the funny side: Train yourself to look for humor in everyday situations, even amidst challenges and difficulties. Adopt a playful and lighthearted attitude towards life's ups and downs, and cultivate a sense of humor that embraces the absurdity and unpredictability of the human experience.

Laugh at yourself: Learn to laugh at yourself and your own foibles, quirks, and mistakes. Humility and self-deprecation not only endear us to others but also help us maintain perspective and humility in the face of adversity. By embracing our imperfections and embracing our imperfections, we can defuse tension and find common ground with others.

Share laughter with others: Cultivate a supportive network of friends and loved ones with whom you can share laughter and levity. Engage in playful banter, share funny stories and jokes, and create opportunities for shared laughter and joy. Laughter is contagious, and sharing it with others strengthens social bonds and fosters a sense of connection and belonging.

Use humor as a coping mechanism: Use humor as a coping mechanism to navigate difficult situations and emotions. Instead of dwelling on negative thoughts or feelings, try to find humor in the absurdity or irony of the situation. By reframing challenges in a more positive light, you can reduce stress and anxiety and foster emotional resilience.

Practice mindful laughter: Practice mindful laughter by immersing yourself fully in the experience of laughter and allowing yourself to savor its joyful, uplifting effects. Pay attention to the sensations, thoughts, and emotions that arise as you laugh, and allow yourself to fully embrace the moment with gratitude and appreciation.

In conclusion, humor is a powerful antidote to life's challenges, offering solace, perspective, and resilience amidst adversity. By embracing humor as a coping mechanism, cultivating a lighthearted attitude towards life, and sharing laughter with others, we can tap into its transformative power to navigate the ups and downs of the human experience with grace, resilience, and joy. As we harness the power of laughter to infuse our lives with levity and laughter, may we discover the boundless capacity for humor and resilience that resides within each of us.

Chapter 24: Seeking balance.

————

In the tumultuous sea of modern life, seeking balance stands as a beacon of stability and harmony amidst the waves of chaos and uncertainty. In this chapter, we explore the importance of balance in turbulent times and offer practical insights on how to find equilibrium between work, life, and relaxation, empowering you to navigate life's challenges with grace and resilience.

The importance of balance in turbulent times.

Balance is not merely a state of equilibrium; it is a dynamic interplay of priorities, responsibilities, and self-care practices that fosters well-being and fulfillment in our lives. Here are several reasons why balance is important, especially in turbulent times:

Physical and mental health: Balance promotes physical and mental health by preventing burnout, exhaustion, and stress-related illnesses. When we maintain a balance between work, life, and relaxation, we replenish our energy reserves and prevent the negative effects of chronic stress on our body and mind.

Fulfillment and well-being: Balance fosters fulfillment and well-being by ensuring that we allocate time and energy to activities that nourish and fulfill us. When we prioritize our health, relationships, and personal interests alongside our work and responsibilities, we experience greater satisfaction and meaning in our lives.

Resilience and adaptability: Balance enhances resilience and adaptability by equipping us with the resources and reserves to navigate life's challenges and uncertainties. When we maintain a sense of balance in our lives, we are better able to cope with setbacks, adjust to change, and bounce back from adversity with greater ease and grace.

How can we find balance between work, life, and relaxation?

Set priorities: Begin by clarifying your priorities and values, so you can make informed decisions about how to allocate your time and energy. Identify the activities, relationships, and pursuits that are most important to you, and use them as a guide for balancing your commitments and responsibilities.

Establish boundaries: Establish clear boundaries around your time, energy, and resources, and communicate them assertively to others. Learn to say no to non-essential tasks or commitments that detract from your well-being, and prioritize activities that align with your values and priorities.

Schedule Regular Breaks: Schedule regular breaks throughout your day to rest, recharge, and rejuvenate. Take short breaks between tasks to stretch, breathe deeply, or engage in mindfulness practices, and take longer breaks during the day to eat nutritious meals, go for a walk, or engage in hobbies and activities that bring you joy.

Practice self-care: Prioritize self-care activities that nourish and replenish your body, mind, and spirit. Make time for exercise, healthy eating, adequate sleep, and relaxation techniques such as meditation, yoga, or deep breathing. Engage in activities that bring you joy and fulfillment, and make self-care a non-negotiable part of your daily routine.

Cultivate flexibility: Cultivate flexibility and adaptability in your approach to work and life, recognizing that balance is not a fixed state but a dynamic process of adjustment and recalibration. Be willing to adjust your priorities and commitments as needed to maintain a sense of balance and well-being in your life.

Seek support: Seek support from friends, family members, or colleagues who can offer encouragement, advice, and assistance in maintaining balance in your life. Share your struggles and challenges openly with others, and don't hesitate to ask for help when needed. Remember that you don't have to navigate life's challenges alone.

In conclusion, seeking balance between work, life, and relaxation is essential for fostering well-being, resilience, and fulfillment in turbulent times. By setting priorities, establishing boundaries, scheduling regular breaks, practicing self-care, cultivating flexibility, and seeking support, we can find equilibrium in the midst of life's chaos and uncertainty. As we embrace the pursuit of balance as a lifelong journey of self-discovery and growth, may we discover the peace, harmony, and fulfillment that come from living a balanced and authentic life.

Chapter 25: The art of letting go.

———

In the intricate dance of life, the art of letting go emerges as a profound practice that frees us from the burdens of the past and opens the door to new possibilities and growth. In this chapter, we explore why letting go is crucial for our mental health and offer practical exercises to promote the gentle release of that which no longer serves us, empowering us to embrace the present moment with clarity and grace.

Why is letting go important for our mental health?

Letting go is not an act of surrender or defeat; rather, it is an act of liberation and empowerment that frees us from the grip of attachment, resentment, and fear. Here are several reasons why letting go is essential for our mental health:

Release of negative emotions: Holding onto past grievances, regrets, or resentments can weigh heavily on our minds and spirits, leading to feelings of anger, bitterness, or sadness. Letting go allows us to release these negative emotions and make space for healing, forgiveness, and inner peace.

Reduction of stress and anxiety: Clinging to worries about the future or regrets about the past can create unnecessary stress and anxiety, preventing us from fully experiencing the present moment. Letting go of the need to control outcomes or dwell on past mistakes allows us to surrender to the flow of life with greater ease and acceptance.

Cultivation of resilience: Letting go fosters resilience by teaching us to adapt to change and embrace uncertainty with courage and grace. When we release our attachment to specific outcomes or expectations, we become more flexible and resilient in the face of life's inevitable ups and downs.

Promotion of self-compassion: Letting go of self-criticism, perfectionism, or unrealistic expectations fosters greater self-compassion and self-acceptance. When we let go of the need to be perfect or to live up to others' standards, we can embrace ourselves with kindness and understanding, acknowledging our inherent worth and dignity.

Practical exercises to promote letting go.

Mindful awareness: Begin by cultivating mindful awareness of your thoughts, emotions, and sensations in the present moment. Notice any attachments or clinging tendencies that arise, and observe them with curiosity and compassion. Allow yourself to let go of any judgments or expectations, and simply be with whatever arises with an open heart and mind.

Journaling: Take time to journal about any thoughts, emotions, or experiences that are weighing heavily on your mind and heart. Write freely and without judgment, allowing your thoughts and feelings to flow onto the page. Notice any patterns or themes that emerge, and consider whether there are any beliefs or attachments that you may be ready to release.

Forgiveness practice: Engage in a forgiveness practice to release any lingering resentments or grievances towards yourself or others. Reflect on any past hurts or conflicts, and consider whether you are willing to forgive yourself or others for any perceived wrongs. Practice offering forgiveness with an open heart and a spirit of compassion, knowing that it is a gift you give yourself as much as to others.

Visualization: Practice visualization techniques to imagine yourself letting go of any attachments or burdens that you may be carrying. Close your eyes and visualize yourself releasing these burdens into the universe, watching them dissolve into the vast expanse of space.

Notice how it feels to let go and surrender to the flow of life, trusting in the wisdom and guidance of the universe.

Gratitude practice: Cultivate a gratitude practice to shift your focus from what you lack to what you have, fostering a sense of abundance and appreciation in your life. Take time each day to reflect on three things you are grateful for, no matter how small or insignificant they may seem. Notice how gratitude shifts your perspective and opens your heart to the blessings that surround you.

In conclusion, the art of letting go is a transformative practice that fosters healing, resilience, and inner peace. By releasing attachments, resentments, and expectations, we create space for healing, growth, and renewal in our lives. As we cultivate the courage and wisdom to let go of that which no longer serves us, may we discover the freedom, joy, and liberation that come from embracing the present moment with clarity and grace.

Chapter 26: The power of forgiveness.

———

In the intricate tapestry of human relationships, forgiveness emerges as a potent force for healing, reconciliation, and liberation. In this chapter, we delve into the profound significance of forgiveness for our emotional health and offer practical insights on how to cultivate forgiveness and move forward with grace and resilience.

Why is forgiveness important for our emotional health?

Forgiveness is not a sign of weakness or capitulation; it is a courageous act of self-empowerment and liberation that frees us from the shackles of resentment, anger, and bitterness. Here are several reasons why forgiveness is crucial for our emotional health:

Release of emotional burdens: Holding onto grudges, resentment, or anger can weigh heavily on our hearts and minds, leading to feelings of bitterness, hostility, and emotional distress. Forgiveness allows us to release these emotional burdens and make space for healing, compassion, and inner peace.

Reduction of stress and anxiety: Carrying the weight of past hurts or grievances can create unnecessary stress and anxiety, preventing us from fully experiencing joy and fulfillment in the present moment. Forgiveness frees us from the grip of the past and allows us to embrace the present with greater ease and acceptance.

Restoration of relationships: Forgiveness is a powerful catalyst for reconciliation and healing in relationships that have been strained or damaged by conflict or betrayal. By extending forgiveness to others and ourselves, we create opportunities for healing, understanding, and renewed connection.

Promotion of self-compassion: Forgiveness fosters self-compassion and self-acceptance by releasing us from the grip of self-criticism, blame, and shame. When we forgive ourselves for past mistakes or shortcomings, we cultivate greater self-compassion and self-love, acknowledging our inherent worth and dignity as human beings.

How can we learn to forgive and move forward?

Cultivate empathy and compassion: Begin by cultivating empathy and compassion towards yourself and others, recognizing that we are all imperfect beings navigating the complexities of life. Practice putting yourself in the shoes of others and seeing the world from their perspective, fostering understanding and empathy for their struggles and challenges.

Practice self-reflection: Take time to reflect on the ways in which holding onto grudges or resentment may be impacting your emotional health and well-being. Notice any patterns or triggers that arise when you think about past hurts or grievances, and consider how forgiveness could benefit your own mental and emotional health.

Shift your perspective: Shift your perspective from seeing forgiveness as a sign of weakness or capitulation to recognizing it as an act of strength and empowerment. Understand that forgiveness is not about condoning or excusing the actions of others but about releasing yourself from the burden of carrying anger and resentment.

Practice forgiveness meditation: Engage in forgiveness meditation practices to cultivate a sense of compassion and forgiveness towards yourself and others. Set aside time each day to sit quietly and reflect on past hurts or grievances, and practice offering forgiveness with an open heart and mind. Visualize yourself releasing any negative emotions or attachments and embracing a sense of peace and liberation.

Seek support: Seek support from friends, family members, or a therapist who can offer guidance and encouragement as you navigate the process of forgiveness. Share your struggles and challenges openly with others, and allow yourself to receive the support and compassion you need to heal and move forward.

In conclusion, the power of forgiveness is a transformative force for healing, reconciliation, and liberation. By cultivating empathy and compassion, practicing self-reflection, shifting our perspective, engaging in forgiveness meditation, and seeking support, we can learn to forgive ourselves and others and move forward with grace and resilience. As we embrace the healing power of forgiveness in our lives, may we discover the freedom, joy, and liberation that come from letting go of past hurts and embracing a future filled with compassion, understanding, and connection.

Chapter 27: The importance of rest.

I n the relentless rhythm of modern life, the importance of rest emerges as a beacon of sanity and rejuvenation amidst the chaos and demands of daily existence. In this chapter, we delve into the profound significance of rest periods for our physical, mental, and emotional well-being. We also offer practical tips for creating rest periods in our daily lives, empowering us to replenish our energy, restore our balance, and reclaim our vitality.

Why are rest periods crucial?

Rest periods are not merely luxuries or indulgences; they are essential components of a healthy and balanced lifestyle. Here are several reasons why rest periods are crucial:

Physical recovery: Rest periods allow our bodies to recover and repair from the stresses and strains of daily life, promoting muscle recovery, tissue repair, and overall physical rejuvenation. Adequate rest is essential for preventing burnout, fatigue, and overuse injuries, and for maintaining optimal physical health and vitality.

Mental rejuvenation: Rest periods provide our minds with the opportunity to recharge and refresh, promoting mental clarity, focus, and creativity. Taking breaks from mental tasks allows our brains to rest and reset, improving cognitive function, memory, and problem-solving abilities.

Emotional well-being: Rest periods are essential for maintaining emotional well-being and resilience in the face of life's challenges and stressors. Taking time to rest and relax allows us to recharge our emotional batteries, reduce stress and anxiety, and cultivate a greater sense of inner peace and balance.

Enhanced productivity: Contrary to popular belief, rest periods are not a hindrance to productivity; they are essential for sustaining high levels of performance and efficiency over the long term. Taking regular breaks from work or other activities allows us to replenish our energy reserves, maintain focus and concentration, and prevent mental and physical fatigue.

Practical tips for creating rest periods in daily life.

Schedule regular breaks: Incorporate regular breaks into your daily schedule to rest and recharge, especially during periods of intense mental or physical activity. Set aside time every hour or two to take a short break, stretch, or engage in relaxation techniques such as deep breathing or mindfulness meditation.

Prioritize sleep: Make sleep a top priority by ensuring that you get an adequate amount of restful sleep each night. Aim for seven to nine hours of sleep per night, and create a relaxing bedtime routine to help you unwind and prepare for sleep. Turn off electronic devices at least an hour before bedtime, and create a calm and comfortable sleep environment free from distractions.

Practice mindful rest: Cultivate the art of mindful rest by engaging in activities that promote relaxation and rejuvenation, such as spending time in nature, practicing yoga or tai chi, or simply sitting quietly and savoring the present moment. Allow yourself to fully immerse in the experience of rest and relaxation, without judgment or expectation.

Set boundaries: Learn to set boundaries around your time and energy, and prioritize activities that nourish and replenish you. Say no to non-essential commitments or obligations that detract from your well-being, and give yourself permission to take time for rest and self-care without guilt or apology.

Disconnect and unplug: Take regular breaks from technology and screens to give your mind and eyes a rest from constant stimulation. Set boundaries around your use of electronic devices, and designate specific times during the day when you will disconnect and unplug from email, social media, and other digital distractions.

Nurture yourself: Make self-care a priority by engaging in activities that nourish and replenish your body, mind, and spirit. Take time each day to do something you enjoy, whether it's reading a book, taking a bath, or spending time with loved ones. Prioritize activities that bring you joy and fulfillment, and make rest and relaxation a non-negotiable part of your daily routine.

In conclusion, the importance of rest cannot be overstated in our fast-paced and hectic world. By prioritizing rest periods in our daily lives and embracing practices that promote physical, mental, and emotional rejuvenation, we can replenish our energy, restore our balance, and reclaim our vitality. As we honor the need for rest and relaxation in our lives, may we discover the profound benefits of rest for our overall health and well-being, and may we cultivate a greater sense of peace, joy, and fulfillment in the process.

Chapter 28: Seeking inner peace.

―――――

In the hustle and bustle of modern life, amidst the cacophony of demands and distractions, the quest for inner peace stands as a beacon of serenity and solace. In this chapter, we explore the profound importance of inner peace and offer practical insights on how to cultivate it amidst the chaos and turmoil of external circumstances.

Why is inner peace desirable?

Inner peace is not merely a fleeting state of tranquility; it is a profound sense of calm, clarity, and contentment that arises from within. Here are several reasons why inner peace is desirable:

Emotional well-being: Inner peace fosters emotional well-being by reducing stress, anxiety, and agitation. When we cultivate a sense of inner peace, we are better equipped to manage our emotions and navigate life's challenges with grace and resilience.

Mental clarity: Inner peace enhances mental clarity and focus, enabling us to make decisions with greater clarity and insight. When the mind is calm and centered, we are able to see things more objectively and respond to situations with wisdom and discernment.

Physical health: Inner peace has been linked to improved physical health, including lower blood pressure, reduced risk of heart disease, and enhanced immune function. By reducing stress and promoting relaxation, inner peace supports the body's natural healing mechanisms and strengthens overall health and vitality.

Fulfillment and joy: Inner peace brings a sense of fulfillment and joy that transcends external circumstances. When we are at peace with ourselves and the world around us, we experience a deep sense of contentment and gratitude for the present moment.

How can we find inner peace even amidst external chaos?

Cultivate mindfulness: Cultivate mindfulness through practices such as meditation, deep breathing, or mindful movement. Bring your awareness to the present moment, noticing your thoughts, emotions, and sensations without judgment or attachment. By cultivating mindfulness, we can find inner peace even amidst the chaos and noise of external circumstances.

Let go of attachments: Let go of attachments to outcomes, expectations, and desires that cause stress and anxiety. Recognize that true peace comes from within and cannot be dependent on external circumstances or the actions of others. Release the need to control or manipulate outcomes and embrace the present moment with acceptance and surrender.

Practice gratitude: Cultivate gratitude for the blessings and abundance in your life, no matter how small or seemingly insignificant. Take time each day to reflect on the things you are grateful for, and express appreciation for the beauty and wonder of the world around you. Gratitude opens the heart to joy and fulfillment, fostering a sense of inner peace and contentment.

Set boundaries: Set clear boundaries around your time, energy, and relationships to protect your inner peace. Learn to say no to activities or commitments that drain your energy or cause stress, and prioritize activities that nourish and replenish you. By honoring your own needs and boundaries, you create space for inner peace to flourish.

Cultivate compassion: Cultivate compassion for yourself and others, recognizing that we are all imperfect beings navigating the complexities of life. Practice empathy and understanding towards yourself and others, and offer kindness and support whenever possible. Compassion opens the heart to love and connection, fostering a sense of inner peace and harmony.

In conclusion, the quest for inner peace is a journey of self-discovery and transformation that offers profound benefits for our emotional, mental, and physical well-being. By cultivating mindfulness, letting go of attachments, practicing gratitude, setting boundaries, and cultivating compassion, we can find inner peace even amidst the chaos and turmoil of external circumstances. As we embrace the journey of seeking inner peace, may we discover the boundless joy, fulfillment, and serenity that arise from living with an open heart and a peaceful mind.

Chapter 29: The power of visualization.

———

Visualization stands as a potent tool in the arsenal of techniques for finding calm and cultivating inner peace amidst life's storms. In this chapter, we'll explore how visualization techniques can aid us in discovering tranquility and offer practical guides for using visualization to foster inner peace.

How can visualization techniques help us find calm?

Visualization harnesses the power of imagination to create mental images and scenarios that evoke feelings of peace, relaxation, and well-being. By engaging our senses and emotions, visualization techniques can help us access a state of deep calm and inner peace. Here's how visualization can aid in finding calm:

Stress reduction: Visualization can help reduce stress by guiding us into a state of relaxation and tranquility. By picturing ourselves in a serene setting or imagining soothing sensations, we activate the body's relaxation response, lowering blood pressure, reducing muscle tension, and calming the mind.

Emotional regulation: Visualization techniques can aid in emotional regulation by helping us manage difficult emotions such as anxiety, anger, or sadness. By visualizing ourselves in a state of calm and peace, we shift our focus away from distressing thoughts and emotions, allowing us to regain a sense of equilibrium and stability.

Mental clarity: Visualization promotes mental clarity by quieting the mind and enhancing focus and concentration. By visualizing clear and vivid images of our goals, aspirations, or desired outcomes, we clarify our intentions and strengthen our resolve, paving the way for greater success and fulfillment.

Positive reinforcement: Visualization can serve as a powerful tool for reinforcing positive beliefs and attitudes. By repeatedly visualizing ourselves experiencing feelings of calm, confidence, and inner peace, we create new neural pathways in the brain that support these positive states, making them more accessible in our daily lives.

Practical guides to visualization for inner peace.

Relaxation visualization: Find a comfortable position and close your eyes. Take a few deep breaths to center yourself, then visualize yourself in a tranquil setting such as a peaceful beach, lush forest, or serene mountaintop. Imagine the sights, sounds, and sensations of this place, allowing yourself to fully immerse in its beauty and tranquility. Feel a sense of deep relaxation and peace wash over you as you breathe deeply and let go of tension with each exhale.

Inner sanctuary visualization: Create a mental sanctuary—a safe and peaceful place that exists within you. Visualize this sanctuary in vivid detail, including elements such as soft lighting, comfortable furnishings, and beautiful natural surroundings. Imagine yourself surrounded by a sense of warmth, safety, and unconditional love. Whenever you feel stressed or overwhelmed, return to this inner sanctuary in your mind's eye to find refuge and solace.

Affirmation visualization: Choose a positive affirmation or mantra that resonates with you, such as "I am calm and centered" or "I trust in the flow of life." Close your eyes and repeat this affirmation to yourself, allowing the words to sink deep into your subconscious mind. Visualize yourself embodying this affirmation, feeling a sense of calm, confidence, and inner peace radiating from within. Repeat this visualization regularly to reinforce positive beliefs and attitudes.

Future self visualization: Visualize yourself in the future as the calm, confident, and resilient person you aspire to be. See yourself navigating life's challenges with grace and ease, responding to situations with wisdom and clarity. Imagine the feelings of peace, fulfillment, and inner harmony that accompany this version of yourself. Use this visualization as inspiration to take positive steps towards embodying your ideal self in the present moment.

In conclusion, the power of visualization is a potent ally on the journey towards inner peace and tranquility. By harnessing the creative power of our minds to conjure images of peace, relaxation, and well-being, we can access a profound sense of calm and inner harmony. As we cultivate a regular practice of visualization, may we discover the boundless potential for peace and serenity that resides within us, waiting to be awakened and embraced.

Chapter 30: The importance of faith and spirituality.

———

In the tumultuous journey of life, amidst the storms of uncertainty and chaos, faith and spirituality stand as guiding lights, offering solace, strength, and serenity to the weary soul. In this chapter, we delve into the profound importance of faith and spirituality in finding calm amidst turbulent times and offer practical insights on how to integrate spiritual practices into daily life.

How can faith or spirituality help us find calm in turbulent times?

Providing a sense of meaning and purpose: Faith and spirituality provide a framework for understanding the deeper meaning and purpose of life, even amidst adversity and uncertainty. Belief in a higher power or spiritual truth can offer solace and comfort, helping us make sense of life's challenges and find meaning in our experiences.

Fostering resilience and hope: Faith and spirituality cultivate resilience and hope by offering a sense of trust and surrender to a higher power or divine plan. When we have faith that everything happens for a reason and that we are supported by a higher power, we can navigate life's challenges with greater courage, resilience, and optimism.

Offering guidance and support: Faith and spirituality offer guidance and support through teachings, scriptures, and spiritual practices that provide wisdom and insight for navigating life's challenges. Spiritual beliefs and practices can offer solace and comfort during difficult times, providing a sense of connection to something greater than ourselves.

Cultivating inner peace and serenity: Faith and spirituality cultivate inner peace and serenity by offering practices such as prayer, meditation, and mindfulness that quiet the mind and open the heart to divine presence. Spiritual practices help us connect with our innermost selves and with the divine, fostering a sense of peace and tranquility amidst the chaos of external circumstances.

Practical ways to integrate spiritual practices into daily life

Establishing a daily spiritual practice: Set aside time each day for a spiritual practice that nourishes your soul and connects you with your faith or spirituality. This could include meditation, prayer, reading sacred texts, or engaging in acts of devotion or service. Consistency is key, so commit to making your spiritual practice a priority in your daily routine.

Practicing gratitude and mindfulness: Cultivate gratitude and mindfulness as spiritual practices that deepen your connection with the present moment and with the divine. Take time each day to reflect on the blessings and abundance in your life, and practice mindfulness by bringing your awareness to the sensations, thoughts, and emotions that arise in each moment.

Seeking community and support: Connect with a spiritual community or support group that shares your beliefs and values, providing encouragement, guidance, and fellowship along your spiritual journey. Attend religious services, spiritual gatherings, or study groups where you can deepen your understanding of your faith or spirituality and connect with like-minded individuals.

Engaging in acts of service and compassion: Practice acts of service and compassion as expressions of your faith or spirituality, reaching out to others in need and offering support, kindness, and love. Volunteer with charitable organizations, participate in community service projects, or simply lend a helping hand to those in need.

Cultivating a spirit of forgiveness and love: Cultivate forgiveness and love as central tenets of your faith or spirituality, recognizing the inherent worth and dignity of every human being. Practice forgiveness towards yourself and others, releasing resentment and anger and embracing love and compassion as guiding principles in your interactions with others.

In conclusion, the importance of faith and spirituality in finding calm amidst turbulent times cannot be overstated. By cultivating faith, resilience, and hope, and integrating spiritual practices such as prayer, meditation, and acts of service into our daily lives, we can find solace, strength, and serenity in the midst of life's storms. As we deepen our connection with the divine and with our innermost selves, may we discover the peace, joy, and fulfillment that come from living in alignment with our highest spiritual truths and values.

Chapter 31: The art of listening.

─────

In the bustling symphony of human interaction, the art of listening emerges as a profound practice that fosters understanding, empathy, and connection. In this chapter, we explore the importance of listening for interpersonal relationships and offer practical insights on how to cultivate the art of listening to find calm amidst the noise of daily life.

Why is listening important for interpersonal relationships?

Listening is not merely a passive activity; it is an active and intentional practice that deepens our connections with others and fosters mutual understanding and respect. Here are several reasons why listening is crucial for interpersonal relationships:

Fostering understanding: Listening fosters understanding by allowing us to truly hear and comprehend the thoughts, feelings, and perspectives of others. When we listen attentively to someone, we validate their experiences and emotions, creating a space for open and honest communication.

Building trust and empathy: Listening builds trust and empathy by demonstrating our genuine interest and concern for the well-being of others. When we listen with empathy and compassion, we create a sense of safety and acceptance that encourages others to open up and share their thoughts and feelings with us.

Resolving conflicts: Listening is essential for resolving conflicts and misunderstandings in relationships. By actively listening to each other's concerns and perspectives, we can identify common ground and work together to find mutually acceptable solutions to our differences.

Strengthening relationships: Listening strengthens relationships by deepening our connections with others and fostering a sense of intimacy and closeness. When we feel heard and understood by others, we are more likely to trust and respect them, leading to stronger and more fulfilling relationships.

How can we learn to listen better and thereby find calm?

Practice active listening: Practice active listening by giving your full attention to the speaker and engaging with them fully in the present moment. Maintain eye contact, nod your head in acknowledgment, and offer verbal and nonverbal cues that you are listening attentively.

Suspend judgment and assumptions: Suspend judgment and assumptions when listening to others, allowing them to express themselves freely without fear of criticism or condemnation. Approach each conversation with an open mind and a willingness to consider perspectives that may differ from your own.

Reflect and clarify: Reflect back what you hear to ensure that you understand the speaker's message accurately. Paraphrase their words, ask clarifying questions, and validate their emotions to demonstrate that you are truly listening and seeking to understand.

Practice empathy and compassion: Practice empathy and compassion when listening to others, acknowledging their feelings and experiences with warmth and understanding. Put yourself in their shoes and imagine how they might be feeling, and respond with kindness and empathy.

Cultivate patience and presence: Cultivate patience and presence in your interactions with others, allowing them the time and space to express themselves fully. Avoid interrupting or rushing the conversation, and instead, practice being fully present and attentive to the speaker's needs and concerns.

Seek feedback and learn from mistakes: Seek feedback from others on your listening skills and be open to learning from your mistakes. Ask for honest feedback on how well you listen and how you can improve, and use this feedback as an opportunity for growth and self-reflection.

In conclusion, the art of listening is a transformative practice that deepens our connections with others and fosters understanding, empathy, and respect in our relationships. By practicing active listening, suspending judgment and assumptions, reflecting and clarifying, practicing empathy and compassion, cultivating patience and presence, and seeking feedback and learning from mistakes, we can learn to listen better and thereby find calm amidst the noise and busyness of daily life. As we cultivate the art of listening in our interactions with others, may we discover the profound joy and fulfillment that come from truly hearing and understanding one another with empathy and compassion.

Chapter 32: Seeking meaningfulness.

In the vast expanse of existence, the pursuit of meaning stands as a beacon of purpose and fulfillment, guiding us on a journey of self-discovery and growth. In this chapter, we delve into the importance of finding meaning in our lives and offer practical strategies for discovering and pursuing our life goals.

Why is it important to find meaning in our lives?

Finding meaning in our lives is not merely a philosophical pursuit; it is a fundamental aspect of human existence that shapes our perceptions, choices, and actions. Here are several reasons why it is important to find meaning in our lives:

Sense of purpose: Finding meaning in our lives gives us a sense of purpose and direction, guiding our choices and actions towards goals that align with our values and aspirations. When we have a clear sense of purpose, we are more motivated, resilient, and fulfilled in our pursuits.

Enhanced well-being: Meaningful pursuits contribute to our overall well-being by fostering a sense of fulfillment, satisfaction, and happiness. When we engage in activities that are meaningful to us, we experience a deeper sense of joy and contentment that transcends external circumstances.

Resilience in adversity: Meaningful goals and aspirations provide a source of strength and resilience in the face of adversity and challenges. When we have a strong sense of purpose and meaning in our lives, we are better equipped to overcome obstacles and setbacks with courage and determination.

Connection and contribution: Finding meaning in our lives enables us to connect with something larger than ourselves and to contribute to the well-being of others and the world around us. Meaningful pursuits often involve acts of service, creativity, or personal growth that benefit not only ourselves but also our communities and society as a whole.

Practical strategies for discovering and pursuing our life goals.

Reflect on values and passions: Take time to reflect on your values, passions, and aspirations, and identify activities and pursuits that align with your deepest desires and interests. Consider what brings you joy, fulfillment, and a sense of purpose, and use this insight to guide your decision-making and goal-setting.

Set meaningful goals: Set meaningful goals that inspire and motivate you to grow and evolve as a person. Choose goals that are challenging yet attainable, and that resonate with your values and aspirations. Break larger goals down into smaller, manageable steps, and create a plan for achieving them over time.

Cultivate self-awareness: Cultivate self-awareness through practices such as mindfulness, meditation, journaling, or therapy, to deepen your understanding of yourself and your innermost desires. Pay attention to your thoughts, feelings, and intuition, and use this awareness to guide your choices and actions towards greater meaning and fulfillment.

Seek inspiration and guidance: Seek inspiration and guidance from mentors, role models, and sources of wisdom and insight that resonate with your values and aspirations. Surround yourself with people who support and encourage your growth and development, and learn from their experiences and perspectives.

Embrace challenges and setbacks: Embrace challenges and setbacks as opportunities for growth and learning, rather than obstacles to be avoided. Approach difficulties with resilience and determination, and view them as stepping stones on your journey towards greater meaning and fulfillment.

Practice gratitude and appreciation: Practice gratitude and appreciation for the blessings and opportunities in your life, no matter how small or seemingly insignificant. Cultivate a mindset of abundance and gratitude, and celebrate your progress and achievements along the way.

In conclusion, the pursuit of meaning in our lives is a transformative journey that shapes our experiences, relationships, and contributions to the world. By reflecting on our values and passions, setting meaningful goals, cultivating self-awareness, seeking inspiration and guidance, embracing challenges and setbacks, and practicing gratitude and appreciation, we can discover and pursue our life goals with clarity, purpose, and joy. As we embark on this journey of self-discovery and growth, may we find meaning and fulfillment in the pursuit of our deepest desires and aspirations, and may our lives be a testament to the power of purpose and meaning to enrich and inspire us all.

Chapter 33: The power of music.

———

Music, with its timeless melodies and harmonious rhythms, possesses a transformative power that transcends language and culture. In this chapter, we explore how music can help us find calm and offer practical tips for using it as a stress relief tool in our daily lives.

How can music help us find calm?

Emotional regulation: Music has the ability to evoke a wide range of emotions, from joy and excitement to tranquility and serenity. By listening to calming melodies or soothing instrumental music, we can regulate our emotions and reduce feelings of stress and anxiety.

Relaxation response: Listening to slow-tempo music with a gentle rhythm can activate the body's relaxation response, leading to decreased heart rate, lowered blood pressure, and reduced muscle tension. This promotes a sense of calm and relaxation throughout the body and mind.

Distraction from negative thoughts: Music provides a welcome distraction from negative thoughts and rumination, offering a mental escape from the stresses and challenges of daily life. Engaging with music allows us to shift our focus away from worries and anxieties, creating a space for peace and tranquility to emerge.

Mindfulness and presence: Music can serve as a powerful tool for cultivating mindfulness and presence, helping us to be fully present in the moment and to immerse ourselves in the rich sensory experience of sound. By listening mindfully to music, we can quiet the chatter of the mind and find refuge in the present moment.

Practical tips for using music as a stress relief tool.

Create a calming playlist: Curate a playlist of calming music that resonates with you and brings a sense of peace and tranquility. Include a variety of genres, from classical and instrumental to ambient and nature sounds, and tailor the playlist to suit your personal preferences and mood.

Practice active listening: Set aside dedicated time each day to engage in active listening to music, focusing your full attention on the sounds, rhythms, and melodies. Close your eyes, take deep breaths, and allow yourself to be fully immersed in the music, letting go of distractions and worries.

Incorporate music into daily routines: Integrate music into your daily routines and activities to enhance relaxation and reduce stress. Listen to calming music while cooking, cleaning, exercising, or commuting, allowing the soothing sounds to accompany you throughout the day.

Experiment with different styles: Experiment with different styles and genres of music to discover what resonates with you and brings you the greatest sense of calm and relaxation. Explore classical compositions, ambient soundscapes, nature sounds, or guided meditation music, and notice how each affects your mood and state of mind.

Use music for meditation and mindfulness: Incorporate music into your meditation and mindfulness practices to deepen your sense of relaxation and presence. Choose music with a slow tempo and gentle rhythm to support your practice, and allow the sounds to guide you into a state of deep relaxation and inner stillness.

Play an instrument or sing: Engage actively with music by playing an instrument or singing, tapping into the creative expression and emotional release that music offers. Whether you're strumming a guitar, playing piano, or singing along to your favorite songs, allow yourself to be fully immersed in the joy and beauty of music-making.

In conclusion, the power of music to calm the mind, soothe the soul, and uplift the spirit is truly remarkable. By incorporating music into our daily lives and using it as a stress relief tool, we can tap into its transformative potential to promote relaxation, mindfulness, and emotional well-being. As we open ourselves to the healing and rejuvenating power of music, may we find solace, inspiration, and joy in its timeless melodies and harmonious rhythms, and may it serve as a source of comfort and strength on our journey towards greater peace and serenity.

Chapter 34: The healing power of nature.

———

Nature, with its vast landscapes, tranquil forests, and awe-inspiring beauty, holds a profound and transformative power over the human psyche. In this chapter, we explore the therapeutic effects of nature on our mental and emotional well-being and offer practical ways to utilize nature to find calm in our lives.

The therapeutic effects of nature on our psyche.

Stress reduction: Spending time in nature has been shown to reduce levels of stress hormones such as cortisol and adrenaline. The serene sights and sounds of natural environments promote relaxation and calm, helping to alleviate feelings of anxiety and tension.

Mood enhancement: Nature has a remarkable ability to uplift our mood and improve our overall sense of well-being. The beauty and tranquility of natural landscapes evoke feelings of awe, wonder, and joy, leading to a more positive outlook on life.

Mental clarity and focus: Immersing ourselves in natural surroundings can sharpen our focus and enhance cognitive function. Nature provides a respite from the constant stimulation and distractions of modern life, allowing our minds to rest and recharge.

Emotional healing: Nature has a soothing effect on our emotions, offering solace and comfort during times of sadness, grief, or loss. The gentle rhythms of nature's cycles remind us of the inherent resilience and beauty of life, fostering a sense of hope and renewal.

Practical ways to utilize nature to find calm.

Spend time outdoors: Make a conscious effort to spend time outdoors in natural settings such as parks, forests, beaches, or gardens. Take leisurely walks, go hiking, or simply sit and soak in the sights and sounds of nature.

Practice mindful observation: Engage in mindful observation of nature by paying close attention to the sights, sounds, and sensations of your surroundings. Notice the colors and shapes of the landscape, listen to the rustling of leaves or the chirping of birds, and feel the warmth of the sun on your skin.

Connect with the elements: Connect with the elements of nature by immersing yourself in activities such as swimming in a lake, feeling the earth beneath your feet, or gazing at the stars on a clear night. Allow yourself to feel a sense of awe and wonder at the beauty and majesty of the natural world.

Engage in nature-based practices: Engage in nature-based practices such as gardening, birdwatching, or nature photography to deepen your connection with the natural world. These activities not only provide a sense of purpose and fulfillment but also offer opportunities for relaxation and contemplation.

Create a nature-inspired sanctuary: Bring the beauty of nature into your home or workspace by incorporating elements such as plants, natural light, or nature-inspired artwork. Create a cozy reading nook by a window with a view of the outdoors, or surround yourself with images of serene landscapes to evoke feelings of peace and calm.

Practice nature-based mindfulness and meditation: Practice mindfulness and meditation in natural settings to deepen your sense of connection with the earth and sky. Find a quiet spot outdoors, close your eyes, and focus on your breath as you listen to the sounds of nature and feel the gentle rhythm of the earth beneath you.

In conclusion, the healing power of nature is a balm for the soul, offering solace, rejuvenation, and renewal to those who seek its embrace. By immersing ourselves in the beauty and tranquility of the natural world and incorporating nature-based practices into our daily lives, we can tap into its transformative potential to find calm, clarity, and inner peace. As we open our hearts to the healing presence of nature, may we find refuge and inspiration in its timeless beauty, and may it serve as a source of comfort and strength on our journey towards greater well-being and wholeness.

Chapter 35: The importance of fitness and movement.

———

In the fast-paced rhythm of modern life, the significance of physical activity and movement cannot be overstated. In this chapter, we delve into how physical activity can help us find calm and offer practical tips for integrating fitness and movement into our daily lives.

How can physical activity help us find calm?

Stress reduction: Physical activity has been shown to reduce levels of stress hormones such as cortisol and adrenaline. Engaging in exercise releases endorphins, neurotransmitters that act as natural mood lifters, promoting feelings of relaxation and well-being.

Mood enhancement: Exercise is known to boost mood and alleviate symptoms of anxiety and depression. The rhythmic movements of physical activity can induce a meditative state, calming the mind and promoting mental clarity and emotional stability.

Energy boost: Regular physical activity increases energy levels and improves overall vitality. Engaging in exercise increases blood flow and oxygen delivery to the brain and muscles, leaving us feeling invigorated and revitalized.

Improved sleep quality: Physical activity has been linked to improved sleep quality and duration. Regular exercise helps regulate the sleep-wake cycle and promotes deeper, more restful sleep, leading to greater feelings of calm and rejuvenation.

Practical tips for integrating fitness and movement into our daily lives.

Find activities you enjoy: Explore different forms of physical activity and find ones that you enjoy and look forward to. Whether it's walking, running, swimming, dancing, or practicing yoga, choose activities that resonate with your interests and preferences.

Set realistic goals: Set realistic and achievable fitness goals that align with your current level of fitness and lifestyle. Start with small, manageable goals and gradually increase the intensity and duration of your workouts as you progress.

Schedule regular exercise sessions: Make physical activity a priority by scheduling regular exercise sessions into your daily or weekly routine. Block out time in your calendar for workouts, walks, or other forms of movement, treating them as non-negotiable appointments with yourself.

Incorporate movement into daily activities: Look for opportunities to incorporate movement into your daily activities, such as taking the stairs instead of the elevator, walking or cycling to work, or doing household chores such as gardening or cleaning.

Mix up your routine: Keep your workouts interesting and engaging by mixing up your routine and trying new activities or exercises. Incorporate a variety of cardiovascular, strength training, and flexibility exercises to keep your body challenged and motivated.

Listen to your body: Pay attention to your body's signals and adjust your exercise routine as needed to prevent injury and avoid burnout. Rest when you need to, and listen to your body's cues for hunger, thirst, and fatigue.

Stay consistent: Consistency is key to reaping the benefits of physical activity. Make exercise a habit by committing to regular workouts and staying consistent with your fitness routine, even on days when you don't feel like it.

Prioritize recovery: Give your body time to rest and recover after intense workouts, allowing your muscles to repair and rebuild.

Incorporate rest days into your exercise routine, and practice relaxation techniques such as stretching, foam rolling, or meditation to promote recovery and reduce muscle soreness.

In conclusion, the importance of fitness and movement in finding calm and promoting overall well-being cannot be overstated. By engaging in regular physical activity and incorporating movement into our daily lives, we can harness the transformative power of exercise to reduce stress, boost mood, and improve sleep quality. As we prioritize our physical health and vitality, may we discover the profound joy, vitality, and peace that come from living in harmony with our bodies and embracing the gift of movement.

Chapter 36: Seeking truth and authenticity.

―――

In a world filled with noise and distractions, the quest for truth and authenticity stands as a beacon of clarity and purpose. In this chapter, we explore why it is important to be authentic and offer insights on how to find our truth and live authentically.

Why is it important to be authentic?

Self-discovery: Being authentic allows us to discover and embrace our true selves, free from the expectations and judgments of others. By acknowledging our strengths, weaknesses, and unique qualities, we cultivate a deeper sense of self-awareness and acceptance.

Genuine connections: Authenticity fosters genuine connections and meaningful relationships with others. When we show up as our true selves, we attract people who resonate with our values and authenticity, leading to deeper connections based on trust, respect, and mutual understanding.

Inner peace: Living authentically brings a sense of inner peace and alignment with our values and aspirations. When we live in accordance with our truth, we experience a profound sense of fulfillment and contentment that transcends external circumstances.

Personal empowerment: Authenticity empowers us to live life on our own terms, free from the constraints of societal expectations and norms. By embracing our authenticity, we reclaim our power and autonomy, allowing us to pursue our passions and dreams with courage and conviction.

How can we find our truth and live authentically?

Self-reflection: Take time for self-reflection to explore your values, beliefs, and aspirations. Ask yourself probing questions about what truly matters to you and what brings you joy and fulfillment. Journaling, meditation, and introspective practices can help facilitate this process of self-discovery.

Embrace vulnerability: Embrace vulnerability as a pathway to authenticity and connection with others. Be willing to show your true self, including your fears, insecurities, and imperfections. Authenticity requires courage to be seen and heard as we truly are, without pretense or façade.

Trust your intuition: Trust your intuition as a guiding force in finding your truth and living authentically. Tune into your inner wisdom and listen to the whispers of your heart and soul. Trust that your intuition knows what is right for you, even if it goes against conventional wisdom or societal norms.

Set boundaries: Set boundaries to protect your authenticity and honor your truth. Be discerning about the people and situations you allow into your life, and learn to say no to anything that compromises your values or integrity. Boundaries are essential for maintaining your authenticity and well-being.

Practice self-expression: Express yourself authentically through creative outlets such as writing, art, music, or dance. Allow your unique voice and perspective to shine through in your creative endeavors, and use them as vehicles for self-discovery and self-expression.

Cultivate self-compassion: Cultivate self-compassion as you journey towards authenticity, recognizing that it is a process of growth and self-discovery. Be gentle with yourself as you navigate the challenges and uncertainties of living authentically, and practice self-love and acceptance along the way.

Surround yourself with authenticity: Surround yourself with people who support and encourage your authenticity, and seek out environments that allow you to be yourself fully. Authenticity thrives in the presence of like-minded individuals who value truth, integrity, and genuine connection.

In conclusion, the quest for truth and authenticity is a sacred journey of self-discovery and self-expression. By embracing our authenticity and living in alignment with our truth, we reclaim our power, cultivate genuine connections, and experience a profound sense of inner peace and fulfillment. As we honor our truth and embrace our authenticity, may we inspire others to do the same, creating a world where each individual is free to shine brightly as their true and authentic self.

Chapter 37: The art of silence.

———

In the cacophony of modern life, the art of silence emerges as a profound practice that offers solace, clarity, and renewal. In this chapter, we explore why it is important to sometimes be silent and offer practical ways to incorporate silence into our daily lives.

Why is it important to sometimes be silent?

> Inner reflection: Silence provides an opportunity for inner reflection and introspection, allowing us to tune into our inner thoughts, feelings, and intuition. In moments of silence, we can cultivate self-awareness, gain insight into our deepest desires and fears, and discern the next steps on our life's journey.

> Mental clarity: Silence fosters mental clarity and focus by quieting the constant chatter of the mind. In the absence of external distractions, we can concentrate more deeply on the task at hand, solve problems more effectively, and tap into our creativity and intuition.

> Emotional regulation: Silence promotes emotional regulation by creating a space for us to process and integrate our emotions. In moments of silence, we can acknowledge and honor our feelings without judgment or distraction, allowing them to flow freely and dissipate naturally.

> Connection with others: Silence deepens our connection with others by fostering attentive listening and empathic understanding. When we listen without the need to fill the silence with words, we create a safe space for others to express themselves authentically and feel truly heard and understood.

Practical ways to incorporate silence into our daily lives.

Morning silence: Start your day with a few moments of silence before diving into the hustle and bustle of daily life. Set aside time each morning for quiet reflection, meditation, or simply enjoying a cup of tea in silence to center yourself and set a positive tone for the day ahead.

Commute silence: Use your daily commute as an opportunity to embrace silence and cultivate mindfulness. Turn off the radio, podcast, or audiobook, and instead, focus on your breath, observe your surroundings, or practice gratitude for the journey.

Nature silence: Spend time in nature to experience the healing power of silence. Take leisurely walks in the woods, sit by a peaceful lake, or simply bask in the beauty of a sunrise or sunset in silence, allowing the sounds of nature to soothe your soul and reconnect you with the natural world.

Mealtime silence: Practice mindful eating by enjoying meals in silence, free from distractions such as television, smartphones, or conversation. Pay attention to the colors, textures, and flavors of your food, and savor each bite with gratitude and awareness.

Evening silence: Wind down at the end of the day with a few moments of silence before bed. Create a calming bedtime ritual that includes activities such as gentle stretching, deep breathing, or journaling in silence to quiet the mind and prepare for restful sleep.

Technology silence: Take regular breaks from technology to disconnect from the constant noise and stimulation of digital devices. Designate periods of time each day or week for digital detoxes, during which you unplug from screens and immerse yourself in silence and solitude.

Social silence: Practice the art of silence in social interactions by listening more and speaking less. Allow pauses in conversation to unfold naturally, and resist the urge to fill them with unnecessary words. Embrace the richness of silence as a powerful form of communication and connection with others.

In conclusion, the art of silence offers a gateway to inner peace, clarity, and connection in an increasingly noisy and distracted world. By embracing moments of silence throughout our daily lives, we can cultivate self-awareness, mental clarity, and deep connections with ourselves and others. As we honor the power of silence to nurture our souls and nourish our spirits, may we find refuge and renewal in its gentle embrace, and may it guide us towards greater wisdom, compassion, and authenticity in all aspects of our lives.

Chapter 38: The importance of gratitude and generosity.

In a world often characterized by hustle and chaos, the virtues of gratitude and generosity shine as beacons of light, offering solace, connection, and inner peace. In this chapter, we explore how gratitude and generosity can help us find calm and offer practical exercises to promote these virtues in our daily lives.

How can gratitude and generosity help us find calm?

Shift in perspective: Practicing gratitude and generosity can shift our perspective from scarcity to abundance, from focusing on what we lack to appreciating what we have. By cultivating gratitude for the blessings in our lives and sharing our abundance with others, we tap into a sense of fulfillment and contentment that transcends material wealth.

Stress reduction: Gratitude and generosity have been shown to reduce levels of stress hormones such as cortisol and adrenaline. When we express gratitude for the kindness of others or engage in acts of generosity, we experience a sense of connection and well-being that counteracts the negative effects of stress and anxiety.

Cultivation of positive emotions: Gratitude and generosity are powerful catalysts for cultivating positive emotions such as joy, compassion, and kindness. When we acknowledge and appreciate the goodness in our lives, we amplify feelings of happiness and satisfaction. Similarly, when we extend kindness and generosity to others, we experience a sense of fulfillment and purpose that uplifts our spirits.

Strengthening of relationships: Gratitude and generosity foster deeper connections and stronger relationships with others. When we express gratitude for the support and love of friends and family, we strengthen bonds of trust and intimacy. Similarly, when we practice generosity towards others, we build a sense of community and belonging that enriches our lives and the lives of those around us.

Practical exercises to promote gratitude and generosity.

Gratitude journaling: Set aside time each day to write down three things you are grateful for. Reflect on the people, experiences, and blessings in your life, no matter how small or seemingly insignificant. Cultivate a sense of appreciation for the abundance that surrounds you.

Random acts of kindness: Perform random acts of kindness towards others without expecting anything in return. This could be as simple as holding the door open for someone, complimenting a stranger, or paying for someone's coffee. Acts of kindness not only benefit others but also bring a sense of joy and fulfillment to the giver.

Volunteer work: Get involved in volunteer work or community service projects that align with your interests and values. Whether it's serving meals at a homeless shelter, tutoring children, or participating in environmental clean-up efforts, volunteering provides opportunities to practice generosity and make a positive impact in the lives of others.

Gratitude meditation: Practice gratitude meditation to cultivate a sense of inner peace and well-being. Find a quiet space, close your eyes, and focus on your breath. With each inhale, imagine breathing in gratitude and appreciation. With each exhale, release any tension or negativity. Allow feelings of gratitude to fill your heart and radiate outward to others.

Express appreciation: Take time to express appreciation for the people in your life who have made a positive impact on you. Write a heartfelt thank-you note, send a thoughtful text message, or simply offer a sincere word of gratitude in person. Let others know how much you value and appreciate their presence in your life.

Practice generosity of spirit: Cultivate a spirit of generosity in all aspects of your life, from sharing your time and resources with others to offering compassion and forgiveness. Approach each interaction with an open heart and a willingness to give freely of yourself, knowing that generosity begets generosity and enriches the lives of both giver and receiver.

In conclusion, the virtues of gratitude and generosity hold the power to transform our lives and the world around us. By cultivating gratitude for the blessings in our lives and extending generosity towards others, we not only find calm and fulfillment within ourselves but also contribute to a more compassionate and harmonious society. As we embrace the practice of gratitude and generosity as guiding principles in our lives, may we create a ripple effect of kindness and compassion that uplifts and inspires others to do the same.

Chapter 39: The power of small joys.

———

In the hustle and bustle of our daily lives, it's easy to overlook the simple pleasures that surround us. However, the power of small joys cannot be underestimated, as they have the potential to bring immense happiness and fulfillment to our lives. In this chapter, we explore why small joys are important for our well-being and offer practical tips for discovering and appreciating them in our daily lives.

Why are small joys important for our well-being?

Cultivating gratitude: Small joys remind us to cultivate gratitude for the abundance of blessings in our lives, no matter how seemingly insignificant. By appreciating the small moments of beauty, kindness, and wonder that surround us, we shift our focus from what is lacking to what is present, fostering a sense of contentment and fulfillment.

Enhancing mindfulness: Paying attention to small joys encourages mindfulness, as it requires us to be fully present and attentive to the present moment. When we savor the small pleasures of life, whether it's a warm cup of tea, a beautiful sunset, or a heartfelt conversation with a loved one, we deepen our awareness and appreciation of life's simple delights.

Boosting mood and well-being: Small joys have a powerful impact on our mood and well-being, lifting our spirits and infusing our lives with joy and positivity. Even brief moments of happiness, such as sharing a laugh with a friend or enjoying a favorite song, can have a profound effect on our overall happiness and resilience.

Building resilience: Embracing small joys builds resilience by providing moments of light and joy amidst life's inevitable challenges and setbacks. When we take time to appreciate the small pleasures that abound in our lives, we cultivate a sense of optimism and hope that sustains us through difficult times.

Practical tips for discovering and appreciating small joys in daily life.

Practice mindful observation: Cultivate a habit of mindful observation by paying attention to the small details and moments of beauty in your surroundings. Notice the colors, textures, and sounds of your environment, and take time to savor the small pleasures that often go unnoticed.

Keep a gratitude journal: Start a gratitude journal to document the small joys and blessings in your life on a daily basis. Take a few moments each day to reflect on what you are grateful for, whether it's a kind gesture from a stranger, a delicious meal, or a peaceful moment of solitude.

Engage in simple pleasures: Make time for simple pleasures that bring you joy and relaxation, such as reading a good book, taking a leisurely walk in nature, or enjoying a favorite hobby. Embrace moments of rest and rejuvenation, and allow yourself to fully immerse in activities that nourish your soul.

Cultivate presence in relationships: Foster meaningful connections with others by being fully present and engaged in your interactions. Practice active listening, genuine curiosity, and heartfelt communication, and take pleasure in the small moments of connection and intimacy that arise.

Find joy in everyday rituals: Infuse your daily routines and rituals with moments of joy and mindfulness. Whether it's brewing a pot of coffee in the morning, tending to your garden, or preparing a meal with loved ones, find joy in the simple acts of daily living and savor the beauty of the present moment.

Express gratitude and appreciation: Express gratitude and appreciation for the small joys in your life by acknowledging and thanking those who contribute to your happiness and well-being. Share words of appreciation with loved ones, colleagues, and strangers alike, and spread kindness and positivity wherever you go.

Embrace imperfection: Let go of the pressure to seek perfection and embrace the beauty of imperfection in your life. Find joy in the messy, imperfect moments that make life rich and meaningful, and celebrate the uniqueness and authenticity of your experiences.

In conclusion, the power of small joys lies in their ability to infuse our lives with happiness, gratitude, and meaning. By cultivating mindfulness, gratitude, and presence, we can discover and appreciate the small pleasures that abound in our daily lives, enriching our well-being and deepening our connection to the beauty and wonder of the world around us. As we embrace the power of small joys to uplift and inspire us, may we find solace, joy, and fulfillment in the simple pleasures that make life truly extraordinary.

Chapter 40: Life as a journey.

———

Life, with its twists and turns, challenges and triumphs, is often likened to a journey—a passage through time marked by moments of joy, sorrow, growth, and transformation. In this chapter, we explore why it is important to view life as a journey and offer insights on how to continue our journey with courage and calm.

Why is it important to view life as a journey?

Perspective and meaning: Viewing life as a journey provides us with a broader perspective and deeper meaning, helping us to see the bigger picture of our existence. By recognizing that life is a continuous journey of growth and discovery, we gain a sense of purpose and direction that guides our choices and actions.

Resilience and adaptability: Embracing life as a journey cultivates resilience and adaptability in the face of challenges and setbacks. Just as a traveler navigates unexpected detours and obstacles on a journey, we learn to adapt to life's uncertainties with courage, flexibility, and perseverance.

Growth and transformation: Life's journey is a process of continuous growth and transformation, marked by experiences that shape and mold us into the people we are meant to become. By embracing the ebb and flow of life's rhythms, we open ourselves to the possibilities of self-discovery, evolution, and renewal.

Appreciation and gratitude: Viewing life as a journey encourages us to appreciate and savor each moment along the way, recognizing the beauty and blessings that surround us. When we approach life with a spirit of gratitude and appreciation, we find joy and fulfillment in the simple pleasures and experiences that enrich our journey.

How can we continue our journey with courage and calm?

Embrace uncertainty: Embrace the uncertainty of life's journey with courage and curiosity, knowing that each twist and turn holds the potential for growth and discovery. Trust in your ability to navigate life's uncertainties with grace and resilience, and embrace the journey with an open heart and mind.

Cultivate inner strength: Cultivate inner strength and resilience to weather life's challenges and setbacks. Practice self-care, mindfulness, and self-compassion to nourish your mind, body, and spirit, and build a foundation of inner strength that sustains you through life's ups and downs.

Stay present: Stay present in the moment and savor the journey as it unfolds, without dwelling on the past or worrying about the future. Practice mindfulness and awareness to anchor yourself in the here and now, and find joy and peace in the simple pleasures and experiences of daily life.

Embrace change: Embrace change as a natural and inevitable part of life's journey, rather than resisting or fearing it. Be open to new experiences, opportunities, and perspectives, and welcome the growth and transformation that come with embracing life's changes with courage and acceptance.

Seek support and connection: Seek support and connection from others who share your journey, and surround yourself with people who uplift and inspire you. Cultivate meaningful relationships and connections that nourish your soul and provide encouragement and support along the way.

Find meaning and purpose: Find meaning and purpose in your journey by aligning your actions and aspirations with your values and passions. Set intentions and goals that reflect your deepest desires and aspirations, and pursue them with courage, determination, and integrity.

In conclusion, life is a journey of growth, discovery, and transformation—a passage through time that unfolds with each step we take. By embracing life as a journey and continuing our journey with courage and calm, we open ourselves to the possibilities of self-discovery, evolution, and renewal. As we navigate life's twists and turns with grace and resilience, may we find joy, fulfillment, and meaning in the journey itself, and may our hearts be filled with gratitude for the precious gift of life and the adventures that await us on the path ahead.

Ending:

As we conclude this journey through the intricacies of finding calm amidst chaos, may we take a moment to reflect on the wisdom gained and the growth experienced along the way. In the tapestry of life, each chapter explored has woven its own thread, contributing to the rich fabric of our existence. From the depths of chaos to the heights of serenity, we have navigated through challenges and triumphs, learning invaluable lessons that have shaped our journey.

As we stand at the threshold of this book's conclusion, let us carry forward the insights and practices gleaned, anchoring them firmly in the soil of our hearts. Let us remember that courage, resilience, and authenticity are not merely concepts to be contemplated, but virtues to be lived each day. Let us embrace the art of silence, the power of gratitude, and the joy of small moments, finding solace and strength in their embrace.

And as we continue on our journey through life, may we walk with courage and calm, knowing that within us lies the power to navigate even the stormiest seas. Let us cherish each step, each breath, each heartbeat, for they are the rhythm of life itself. And may the path ahead be illuminated by the light of our own inner wisdom and the grace of the universe, guiding us ever onward towards the shores of peace and fulfillment.

With gratitude for the journey shared and the discoveries made, let us bid farewell to these pages, knowing that the journey continues, both within us and beyond. May we carry the lessons learned and the love shared into the world, becoming beacons of light and sources of inspiration for all those we encounter along the way.

For in the end, it is not the destination that matters most, but the journey itself—the winding path of discovery, growth, and transformation that leads us ever closer to the truth of who we are and the beauty of all that we can become. And so, with hearts full of gratitude and minds filled with possibility, let us embrace the journey, wherever it may lead.